Forming a Moral Community

A Resource for Healthcare Ethics Committees

Bioethics Consultation Group
Berkeley, California

Design by Eric Olsen and Vi McFall
Typeset in Palatino by Eric Olsen
Cover design by Pope Graphics
Printed by General Printing, Berkeley, California

The Bioethics Consultation Group Inc. shall not be liable for errors contained herein or for consequential damages in connection with the furnishing or use of this material. Legal, medical and other comments are presented for educational purposes only. Professional advice should be obtained for specific cases.

ISBN # 1-882674-00-6

Acknowledgement

This new edition of *Forming a Moral Community* is the work of many hands; in particular, I wish to thank all of the people who have made up the "moral community" of the ethics committees with which we have worked over the last ten years, including Brian Saunders, M.D., and Peggy Treat, R.N., who developed the preamble and ritual section of our methodology and added a uniquely important dimension to case review. All of these healthcare professionals, community members, patients and their families, have all contributed from their life experience and their wisdom.

Experience alone will not make a useable manual, however; the thinking through and the articulation of the theory, and especially of our methodology, has been formulated by our professional staff and consultants: Sharon Deehan, Laurie Zoloth Dorfman, Angela O'Connell, John Paris, S.J., Susan Rubin, and Stanley Watson.

Special thanks to our editor, Eric Olsen, who has really been the midwife for our first born. Finally, we need to thank Jean and Charles Thompson for their infinite patience with this process of gestation, and for all their practical help.

John D. Golenski, S.J.

LOCATOR GUIDE

Establishing the IEC

Issues relevant to establishing an IEC are covered in the sections listed below.

Initial Organizational Meetings

The first meetings often set the tone for the committee's future. Refer to the following sections for assistance initiating the committee.

Education and Orientation

Committees need both formal and didactic input from experts and the commitment and involvement of self-education. The following sections assist in both.

Ethical Theory

Development of Policies and Protocols

Institutions usually want guidelines for commonly occurring ethical dilemmas. Refer to the following for advice on responding to this need.

Appendices

Case Review Skills

The heart of the IEC's work is reflection on specific ethical questions. Guidelines for developing this skill can be found in the following.

Appendices

Section Three: Methodology

Evaluation and Continued Education

A committee's continued viability depends on its capacity to respond to the demands of the clinical environment. The following sections provide advice in this regard.

Appendices

INTRODUCTION

INTRODUCTION

During the past decade, we've seen the notion of the institutional ethics committee (IEC) grow from a rather outlandish idea to a national movement....

T his handbook is intended for use in the establishment and initial training of ethics committees, and represents a distillation of our experience of nearly a decade helping to establish and train over 200 ethics committees nationwide in a host of settings from large HMOs to university hospitals to church-affiliated hospitals to small community hospitals to hospices.

During the past decade, we've seen the notion of the institutional ethics committee (IEC) grow from a rather outlandish idea to a national movement, most recently verified by the Joint Commission's (JCAHO) Patient's Rights Standards, which require healthcare institutions to have established mechanisms for addressing ethical issues in patient care.

Driving the growing need for ethics committees with clinical case consultation capabilities is the clash between the right of Americans to establish prior directives — verified by the recent Danforth Amendment (see appendix) — and medical science's expanding capability to preserve even the most tenuous of lives. No longer are caregivers, patients and families asking what *can* we do, but rather what *should* we do, and in such situations well-meaning, caring men and women will often differ about what is "right" or "best."

By their very nature, such questions about what should be done, especially when lives hang in the balance, have no easy answers. Through experience, we've come to believe the best approach to resolving conflicts of values and ethical dilemmas is a "mixed model" approach involving a well-functioning ethics committee and coaching by an expert ethics consultant.

It's our belief that the heart of the process of ethical consultation is the committee. While ethics consultants can provide needed expertise in specific cases, and while in-house experts can provide valuable "curbside" consultations during rounds, the committee process is crucial to the kind of clinical work that is increasingly demanded by patients, their families, government, and the general public.

Ethical dilemmas are a matter of legitimate differences of opinion among people around a moral choice (the very existence of an ethical dilemma implies that more than one perception of value is involved). Ethical reflection is a process for resolving conflicting moral visions and claims, not simply a matter of applying clinical competence or technical expertise. Thus we believe that the best way to resolve such dilemmas is in a forum that is interdisciplinary and involves representatives from all clinical units as well as representatives from the community the institution serves.

The differing viewpoints provided by such a multidisciplinary approach ensure that every option is explored. With fresh minds working together, a "synergy" develops that helps everyone rank and weigh his or her values to single out those that are most critical to the issues in the balance, helping to ensure the most thoughtful decisions possible.

As a moral community, a well-functioning IEC provides a new model, a new *modus operandi*, for resolving tensions and values conflicts through a sense of collaboration and mutuality.

You'll find that the heart of this handbook is the Bioethics Consultation Group *methodology*. Just as we firmly believe in the importance of the committee process in resolving ethical dilemmas, we also find that a well-defined *methodology* is central to that process. A methodology guarantees that similar cases are treated similarly, that practitioners attend to all the aspects of the case that should be considered, and that the quality of the committee's work from case to case is consistent. A methodology also amplifies the members' capacity to learn from their experience and develop a transmissible knowledge base.

The BCG methodology has developed out of our experience in a variety of clinical settings. Over the years, we've refined the methodology with the help of ethics committees and committee members around the country, and we and they have found it to be the most effective methodology for working through a case consultation.

We present this handbook now because hospitals and other healthcare institutions around the nation will be faced with the necessity of creating IECs in response to both legal and social pressures. We know the methodology outlined in this handbook works, and works well. The methodology is not a fixed process however; rather, it is constantly being reviewed and refined in an ongoing effort to keep pace with changing values and a changing healthcare environment. We welcome and encourage your suggestions and comments. □

GETTING STARTED

COMMITTEE MEMBERSHIP

The success of an institutional ethics committee will depend on three key decisions made at the outset about its membership: (1) collaborative leadership; (2) diversity of membership; and (3) community members.

Collaborative Leadership

Our experience teaches us that co-chairs are most effective, particularly when one is a physician and the other a nurse, and preferably a nursing manager.

Such joint leadership provides a model of the collaborative practice which is crucial to good ethical reflection and decision-making. We often describe the IEC as a "moral community," that is a community of thoughtful, well-intentioned men and women who are reflecting and working together to make sure that ethical questions about patient care are addressed and resolved. The mutual respect members within this moral community have for one another's differences, and the example they set as a community, may assist in resolving conflicts just as much as the content of their discussions.

In a very real sense, the co-chairs of an IEC — usually a physician and nurse working together — will set the tone for this community, and mentor the collaborative relationship to the rest of the committee and to the clinical community. Ideally, in their role as co-chairs of an IEC, the physician and nurse co-chairs will work together as peers, thus guiding the other IEC members in the transition from the normal hierarchical roles in the clinical setting to the collaboration necessary for the IEC to work.

The Physician Co-Chair: Having a physician as a co-chair sends the clear message to other physicians that their interests will be represented. A common physician objection to ethics committees, and one that any committee will have to manage from day one if it's to function, is physicians' typical fears that the committee will function as a policing agency or a quality assurance mechanism, reviewing cases and second-guessing medical decisions (we'll deal with this objection in more detail in the section of common objections to ethics committees, beginning on page 23). An effective physician co-chair can put this fear to rest at the outset.

Be careful in selecting the physician co-chair; he or she should be one who carries some "weight" with the medical staff, someone who is recognized as a statesman. What do we mean by "weight" or statesmanship? While these terms seem imprecise, the qualities they indicate are recognizable in the right contexts. In a medical staff meeting, for example, when the "statesman" begins to speak, others stop talking and listen. This person also makes sense when speaking, and can exert positive leadership in conflict.

A physician with "weight" is someone who tends to forge consensus in meetings around key issues, rather than dividing the medical staff or focusing on trivial or marginal issues; this person will have an implicit understanding of the political proces, and a talent for it.

The ideal physician co-chair may also be a big admitter to the hospital, or someone on whom subspecialists depend for referrals. He or she, in other words, will have some economic clout around the hospital.

Generally, the candidate for the role of physician co-chair will be someone from primary care, an internist, for example, or someone from a specialty such as cardiology or

Be careful in selecting the physician co-chair; he or she should be one who carries some "weight" with the medical staff, someone who is recognized as a statesman.

pulmonary medicine who spends time in the hospital. Less often, he or she will be a pediatrician or family practice specialist, and rarely a surgeon. Of course, these aren't hard and fast rules, merely guidelines.

While it may be easy to spot the physician with these qualities of statesmanship and leadership, it won't be as easy to find a physician with these qualities plus the time to do the considerable work that's necessary if the committee is to function well. One answer to this particular problem is simple: pay the physician co-chair for his or her time.

This is a radical notion, to be sure, but as healthcare is structured today, with most physicians depending on billable hours for their livelihoods, they won't have much time for such things as ethics committees, or if they do, it'll be in the early mornings or late evenings. However much they like the idea of being involved with an IEC, they'll have to deal with the economic realities of their practice lives. If the hospital or other institution wants a quickly developed, fully-functioning ethics committee without wasting time and energy, the easiest, most direct method is to pay for the time of the physician co-chair; the payback will far outweigh the costs.

There is one caveat, however; once you pay the physician for his or her time, there is the danger the other medical staff may see this individual as working in the interests of the institution, not those of the committee or the medical staff; the physician co-chair must have enough *dignitas* among the physicians to prevent this, which gets back to the importance of selection at the outset. The other co-chair, most likely a nurse, is almost always an employee of the institution and thus will need release time from regular duties to carry out the duties of co-chair.

An additional challenge will be finding someone with

the "people skills" necessary to chair a committee effectively, or who is willing to learn these skills. We've seen many committees with physician co-chairs who are quite energetic, and very knowledgeable about ethics, who simply don't know how to run a meeting. It can be disastrous.

Fortunately, these are skills that can be learned, and there's no shortage of books, videos and seminars about running meetings.

The Nurse Co-Chair: The other co-chair should be someone who understands the necessity for a collaborative working relationship. By virtue of their training and professional experience, nurses are ideal for a leadership role, and in particular, nursing managers.

This isn't an absolute requirement, however; non-nurses can work just as well. But as members of the committee and as part of the committee leadership, nurses can give voice to the concerns and views of the central part of the healthcare team. Because nurses are the ones who must execute care decisions, and because they're exposed to considerable stress when conflicts between these decisions and their own values occur, nurses often are first to notice, and refer, such cases to the ethics committee. Nurses are in a position to closely observe and evaluate the outcomes of decisions that are made about a patient's care as they evolve over time, and which affect not only the patient, but the patient's family and other members of the healthcare team.

In our experience, nursing managers are ideal as co-chairs since they often have access to resources such as clerical and office support that staff nurses and physicians do not, and such support can contribute enormously to the smooth functioning of the committee. Nursing managers also have more "clout" with the nursing staff than individual staff nurses, and perhaps most importantly, a nursing manager co-chair can give a sense to other nurses that they'll be protected when they raise ethical issues. Fear of reprisal is a genuine fear among many nursing staffs, and can hamper the workings of an IEC. For this reason alone, a nursing manager co-chair can play a major role in assuring the effectiveness of the IEC.

In our experience, nursing managers also tend to understand that they have to deal with physicians just as much as with other nurses. There's more risk that staff nurses will either view the IEC as an opportunity to vent their frustrations with the medical staff, or sit mutely as the physician co-chair directs the IEC's discussion.

In choosing a nursing manager as co-chair, take care to find someone who can understand and be sympathetic to the many conflicting interests that typically burden physicians, such as when the physician's own sense of what's appropriate conflicts with the patient's demands and expectations. The co-chair should also understand and be sympathetic to the simple hectic realities of a clinical setting, in which the physician may have discussed these issues at length with the patient and family, but not yet with the nursing staff, simply because of lack of time.

Other Members

How Many? The ideal number of members for an ethics committee is 12 to 20, depending on the size of the institution and the complexity of cases they treat. There's no "quorum" for an IEC meeting, but since an IEC's role is advisory, not deliberative, more rather than fewer members benefit the IEC by contributing to the richness of perspectives brought to bear on a particular problem. A measure of a good IEC is the regular presence of all or most members; likewise, attendance is a primary indicator of a member's commitment and interest, and members who miss meetings frequently shouldn't be on the committee.

Subcommittees: Should members be divided into specialized subcommittees? We'll discuss this question in more detail in the appendix. Briefly, our experience tells us that task-oriented subcommittees work well; these would include a subcommittee to develop policies and guidelines, and a permanent education subcommittee to develop programs for the IEC itself, as well as the institution and community.

There are pros and cons to having a special subcommittee for case consultation, as opposed to a structure in which all members are involved. Some will argue that case consultation is so specialized that you need a subcommittee of individuals with this particular expertise, and the commitment to give it the necessary time. Others argue that the other committee members won't have the opportunity to develop the skills and experience for case consultation, and will be less helpful in full committee meetings. A workable compromise is a rotating subcommittee which allows *all* IEC members to participate over time, though our experience suggests that consultation by the whole IEC is best.

Tenure: We advise against limits on tenure for IEC members. An IEC is not a typical rotating committee for the medical staff, but rather, as we said above, a "moral community." For that community to form and grow and develop the expertise it needs to address complex ethical

subcommittees

tenure

questions, members must be able to participate with no limits set on their service. There's a practical aspect to this as well; the cost of forming an IEC and training its members is not inconsiderable. Also, the normal attrition of members will provide sufficient opportunities for "new blood" without threatening the solid base of experience necessary for a mature committee.

Proportional Representation: However the IEC is structured, membership should reflect a roughly proportional representation of the units that will likely feed cases to the committee; for example, individuals from the tertiary care units, the intensive care nursery, a residents' program — if there is one — and of course a number of staff nurses, are all essential.

A good mix of gender is important, as is a simple majority of physicians, because of the implied protection against subpoena and discovery in most states if the committee is a medical staff committee (see page 16). Ancillary professions must also be represented on the committee, with at least one and perhaps two or more representatives from the social services, and possibly someone from the institution's chaplaincy, if there is one, and if he or she is at all familiar with clinical issues, which isn't always the case. Other care-giving professions may also be represented, as appropriate to the specific institution.

An Ethical Perspective: While seeking proportional representation, however, care must be taken that members are chosen who are perceived by the staff of the institution as representing an ethical perspective. These men and women are easy to spot. Their sensitivity to ethical issues often becomes evident in case committee meetings and ad hoc clinical reviews or interdisciplinary rounds, when you consistently hear them asking questions of an ethical nature (e.g., the dietitian mixing food for a comatose patient on a feeding tube may ask if a decision has been made that feeding is in the patient's best interest; the pharmacist preparing pain medications for a terminal patient may ask if caregivers, in their concern to avoid euthanasia, are prescribing enough; the social worker in touch with the patient's family may often bring up issues the physicians and nurses haven't noticed.)

Such men and women will tend to have an identifiable position or moral stance, so some artful judgments must be made to ensure a richness and diversity of such outlooks among committee members, rather than homogeneity. Diversity will help guarantee that important questions will be asked.

You do want people who are independent of mind and some who will assume the "devil's advocate" position in IEC deliberations, who will ask, "Yes, but, have you considered *this*?" By their questioning, these men and women will tend to move the IEC to deeper reflection; they're a structural mechanism protecting against "group-think."

On the other hand, you don't want extreme radical positions. In any group, there's a "bell curve" of opinion; an IEC, ideally, will draw from the great middle, where there is considerable variation and diversity; if the IEC is allowed to be polarized by the extremes, the committee will be paralyzed by intractable conflict (please see section on non-radical positions for more detail on this point).

extreme radical

positions

We've outlined a rather complex prescription for membership here: proportional representation, members with diverse ethical perspectives and non-radical positions.

Those choosing committee members will have to try to seek some balance between proportional representation and the "wisdom" of members, not that one excludes the other. In a sense, what ought to be sought is a situation rather like that of the Senate and the House, with the House proportionally determined, and the Senate representing "wisdom," at least ideally.

The realities of the available staff from which committee members can be chosen will of course ultimately determine the nature of the committee itself, and whether it leans more toward proportional representation, or more toward "wisdom."

Special Considerations

Community Membership: We cannot emphasize enough the importance of community representation on the Ethics Committee; these individuals are key to the committee's functioning and success for two reasons:

One, it's vitally important to have someone on the committee who can represent, from a non-professional viewpoint, the common values of the community the institution serves. When a patient is admitted to a hospital, for example, he or she and the family in essence enter a pre-existing community with its own distinctive values, not their own; they live by the hospital's rules. One often hears hospital personnel refer to "the house"; it's a peculiar term to use about a hospital, and clearly creates a distinction between the patient and community, and the hospital itself. The presence of community members on the Ethics Committee helps keep institutional representatives honest, helps to relax this barrier between institution and community, and offers a fresh connection with the prevailing values of the community.

The other reason we feel community members are so important is that the other committee members — the professional caregivers — tend to take the committee much more seriously when they know they're under scrutiny by someone from the community; this prevents the committee from degenerating into little more than a discussion club for "insiders".

Community members must not be viewed as "defective" professionals; nor is their role to be just one more voice in the hospital's phalanx of professionals. Rather they're there to voice the concerns specifically of non- professionals. By asking ingenuous questions, they provide an opportunity for others on the committee to examine their own assumptions and biases.

In order for community members to function effectively, however, they must be included in the process of committee formation from the very beginning. A favorite ploy of committee chairs who are opposed to community membership is to invite community members onto the committee only after the other members have received their training. This effectively prevents community members from knowing what the others know, so they're always outsiders. Community members must be selected at the beginning of the committee's life, and they must go through the training everyone else goes through; moreover, if they're not particularly familiar with the clinical setting, then they should be provided with an additional medical/institutional orientation designed specifically for community members prior to committee training.

Who should be selected from the community to serve as

members? In general, it's helpful if they're prominent members of their community, and if they have some familiarity with the clinical setting; ideally, they ought to combine some clinical savvy with involvement in the community.

We've found that benefits managers of large corporations are extremely helpful because they have a good understanding of healthcare. Older volunteers are also often experienced clinically. Other possible members, with either some clinical experience, or some prominence in their communities, include school board members, PTA members, special education teachers, and parents of children with disabilities. Hospital trustees or members of the institutional board of directors are another possibility, though with some reservations; trustees with a financial interest — contractors who have or have had construction contracts with a hospital, for example — should be excluded.

Clergy: While a member of the institution's own chaplaincy can serve as a member of the ethics committee, providing he or she has some familiarity with the clinical setting, be extremely cautious about inviting clergy from outside; representation of one denomination or faith can arouse the ire of others not represented. In our heterogeneous society, in other words, opening the door to one member of the clergy is usually viewed as differentially excluding others.

Administrator: An institutional administrator should be on the committee, perhaps at the vice president level to provide administrative liaison. However, in most cases, the CEO should not be on the IEC. Many CEOs have a long-term interest in ethical questions; they like the committee process and want to be part of it, but their presence dampens discussion. With rare exceptions, CEOs will uninten-

____

clergy

____

administrator

tionally shift the ground of case deliberation to an institutional focus. They don't want this to happen, but unfortunately there's little they can do about it.

An Attorney Member: Under no circumstances should the in-house counsel sit on the IEC. It's an absolute conflict of interest; the in-house counsel can't look after the institution's interests while considering ethical questions of patient care.

But it is helpful if you can find a community attorney who does not do business with the institution, who has a personal interest in ethical questions and the law, and who has some expertise to offer the committee. Such individuals are rare, however, and in their absence, it would be best to contract on a consulting basis with an attorney somewhere in the vicinity whose practice includes these kinds of issues.

If no suitable attorney exists in your community, the in-house counsel may be used on an ad hoc basis once deliberation is over. Great caution must be exercised in this regard (please see "Methodology" for more on this).

Professional Ethicist: A professional ethicist, if such exists in the community, should be on the committee as an external consultant to facilitate clinical case review and provide education.

A professional ethicist should not be the chair of the committee, however. Rather, she or he should be viewed as "a specialty coach," someone with a defined role who attends meetings and is available to the participants in the process, but who is never viewed as the "expert" who tells others what to do. Like a coach, the professional ethicist is at the "game," but doesn't "carry the ball."

Non-radical Positions: The fact an IEC exists, and that cases come before it, means there can be fundamental disagreements about what is best; if everyone agreed all the time, there'd be no need for such committees.

Thus the effectiveness of the IEC derives from the richness and diversity of views of its members; homogeneity of viewpoint must be avoided at all costs. This is essential if the committee is to function well and bring to bear on a question of patient care as many perspectives as possible. The co-chairs of an IEC will understand it's their role to invoke these differing views, to get as complete a picture of the situation as possible before the process of deliberation begins.

Likewise it's crucial that the men and women on the IEC understand that there are differences of ethical positions in the world; they should be people with strongly held views, but who can still accept the fact that those who differ with them are also responsible, intelligent human beings, and that differing views can come from differing experience, training, philosophy, theology, and simply seeing the consequences of actions.

Individuals with positions that are so radical they can't consider a case on the particular merits of that case, and who are unwilling to accept the notion that those who differ with them are equally well-intentioned, will be of limited value to an IEC; the committee will end up spending all of its time managing the extreme individual, rather than reflecting on the case at hand.

A case coming before an IEC will likely pose enormously complex and difficult questions. Each case is a dilemma involving real people whose lives are not subject to another's political or philosophical stance. Individuals holding radical positions will not be of much use in deciding what's best, in that particular case, if they mistake the case at hand as only an example of a political or philosophical question, or who view the case as a platform for their own political positions, and thus are unable to reflect on the moral choices presented by the specific case.

On the other hand, persons holding radical positions would be welcome if they can present their positions as they bear on the *particular* case at hand. Then their views would not only be germane to the discussion, but an important part of it. ☐

CONFIDENTIALITY, RECORDING

T here are three specific layers of record keeping that must be considered by an IEC, and decisions made at the outset by the committee about record keeping will have an impact on committee functioning thereafter.

These three layers are: (1) routine, administrative reporting to whatever entity "oversees" IEC operations; (2) reporting to the physician, nurse, or other party who requests an IEC deliberation; and (3) reporting to the IEC itself, for review and education.

Confidentiality: We cannot overemphasize the importance of confidentiality at every level of reporting. Whatever record keeping is done should fall under the fundamental principle of confidentiality. IEC organizers, leadership, and members, and institution staff and administrators must understand that IEC deliberations are *absolutely* confidential. Confidentiality is the foundation of the trust on which all IEC activities are built; without total adherence to the principle of confidentiality, the IEC cannot function.

The term "report" is an unfortunate term, since it implies broad distribution. We'll use the term throughout with considerable reservations, and with the understanding that any "reporting" done in the context of IEC deliberations is carried out within the requirements of the strictest confidentiality.

Administrative Reporting: One of the issues committee organizers often spend hours worrying about is whether the IEC should be a subcommittee of the administration of the board, or of the Medical Staff Executive Committee.

In our experience it makes absolutely no practical difference whatsoever, but there are some perceptual realities IEC organizers will have to face, such as the concerns of the medical staff. Physicians at the outset will usually express the fear that the IEC will discuss their cases, that they'll be second-guessed, and in the case of litigation, that opposing attorneys will subpoena IEC records and those records will be used against them.

In our opinion, this fear is absolutely unfounded, and we feel that in fact quite the opposite is true: a physician who goes through the process of requesting deliberation by an IEC is in an immensely better situation should litigation ensue; that physician is much better protected when he or she has consultative support. Moreover, we believe that the well-functioning IEC can greatly reduce the risk that litigation will ever occur by helping to resolve conflicts before they reach a point of volatility. This is a view shared by other ethicists and health-law attorneys.

...a physician who goes through the process of requesting deliberation by an IEC is in an immensely better situation should litigation ensue....

But it's hard to convince the medical staff of this at the outset, and IEC organizers can expect medical staff to demand that the IEC be a subcommittee of the Medical Staff Executive Committee. Laws in most states protect IEC records from subpoena if the IEC reports to the Medical Staff Executive Committee, and if a simple majority of members are physicians. Thus it's often easier for the IEC be so constituted, with a simple majority of physicians as members. But again, this is simply an arrangement to allay fears; in our experience, it will have no impact whatsoever on IEC operations.

There is one caveat, however: in some states, there's a problem having a non-physician as the co-chair of the IEC if the committee reports to the Medical Staff Executive Committee. Be sure to check with legal counsel in your area about local statutes; if this is a concern, the simplest solution is to refer to the co-chair as a "vice-chair" on any official reports.

Whether the IEC becomes a subcommittee of the Medical Staff Executive Committee or of the administration, the executive to whom the IEC "reports" must make a fundamental commitment in writing in a mission statement for the IEC that the IEC will be allowed to do its work without influence and intrusion, that the IEC exists as an *independent* forum, and that, again, the principle of confidentiality is absolute.

IEC reports to whatever agency oversees its operations — the Medical Staff Executive Committee, the Board, or the administration — should be as generic as possible, reporting simply who attended and what and how many cases were reviewed.

Reports to the Referring Party: This document is generated at the end of the meeting, and it's for the physician, nurse or other individuals who referred the case to the IEC. Please refer to "Methodology" for a more detailed discussion of the specific reports to referring parties. In general, these reports answer the question being asked in the referral. They can go into the patient's chart if the physician requests this, but *only* upon the physician's request.

For the IEC's Own Education: This third type of report goes into the IEC's own casebook, for use *only* by members of the IEC. This is an internal report kept for members to review. These reports can also serve as the basis for an annual report. These documents should be written with future members in mind. In a sense, they are the living "archives" of the IEC. They will serve as the basis for orienting future members to the case review history of the IEC. □

OBSTACLES

R esistance to IECs is not uncommon; knowing likely objections to their formation and existence in advance can help smooth the way.

Money and Resources: The issue of money can be a major obstacle, especially in this era of rising healthcare costs and declining reimbursements. One of the first objections to the formation of an IEC is likely to be the costs of training, time away from the job, a meeting space, and materials as mundane as copy paper and file folders, books, and so on.

In fact, a well-functioning IEC can be of significant financial benefit to the institution through preventive conflict resolution and by facilitating more appropriate utilization decisions. Another benefit, one which can't be measured directly in dollars and cents, but which is nonetheless significant, is increased physician tie-in to the institution, something healthcare organizations these days are working hard to create. The bottom line is that well-run IECs are a very good investment.

Medical Staff Objections: As discussed previously, there will be considerable concern among the medical staff that the IEC could expose them to greater risk of litigation, and that the IEC will simply be another policing agency "second-guessing" their practice of medicine.

Again, when a case has been reviewed prospectively by a mature, well-functioning IEC, this can be a primary protection against malpractice litigation. IECs tend to mitigate and relieve nurse/physician conflicts before they explode into truly divisive conflicts, making the physician's life easier. Finally, in this era of growing demands by patients for autonomy, IECs can help the physician meet the patient's wishes while being protected from possible litigation (Please see "Legal Issues".)

Another more subtle objection is the view of some physicians, particularly in more traditional areas of the country, or those associated with academic institutions, that what we call an "ethical dilemma" is really a clinical problem, a puzzle which the physician, and the physician alone, can solve by exercising his or her training, skills, experience and personal moral values. When presented with the possibility of an ethics committee review, these physicians will ask, "What do I need with a collection of people not trained in my area to tell me how to solve what is in fact a clinical dilemma?"

An ethical dilemma is not simply a clinical question, however. It is not a technical problem, but a values dispute or question embedded in a clinical case. Such values disputes exist among a community of people comprised of physicians, nurses, administrators, the institution, the general community, the patient and the patient's family. The very process of reflection in the committee is the important goal here, not solely the solution of a particular puzzle about what to do.

Crafting a useful recommendation to help resolve the ethical dilemma will require members to transcend their normal roles in the healthcare setting; they will need to expand their perspective and bring their own moral intuitions and experiences in life to bear on the dilemma, in addition to their clinical expertise. Certainly a capacity for empathy, for moral imagination and for clear- headed thinking about broad human questions will be at least as important as clinical expertise in this setting. Understanding this requires a fundamental shift in perspective.

The Nurses' Objections: These are perhaps the most difficult with which to deal. Nurses may dismiss the IEC as "just
another doctor committee, another way they'll control us
and not hear our voices." In a committee that functions well,
precisely the opposite is true; a good IEC will empower the
nurses and give a form to their voices. However, convincing
nurses of this before the fact is difficult, but as mentioned
above, a nursing manager co-chair can do much to allay the
fears of the nursing staff and assure them they can speak
out, and be protected when they do so.

Lawyer's Objections: Just as some physicians will tend to
view ethical dilemmas as clinical puzzles to be solved by
their own decisions, lawyers may tend to view these dilemmas as legal problems requiring the application of their
specific skills, rather than requiring a forum for differing
perspectives. Lawyers may tend to feel that with their
expertise and knowledge of precedential cases and insights
about what a judge or jury will say, or their skills in using
the particularities of statutory and case law to protect their
client, any so-called "ethical dilemma" can be solved.

The counter to this objection is clear; while some ethical
dilemmas reflect themselves in court decisions, court decisions don't give us a method for making decisions, only
guidance in some case instances. As in dealing with the
physicians' objections, dealing with the lawyers' objections
to the existence of an IEC requires a fundamental shift in
perspective.

Obstacles to Ongoing Functioning

The benefits of an IEC are proportional to how well-run it is; throughout this discussion on the establishment and "growing" of an IEC, we've referred again and again to the "well-run" or "mature" IEC. There are several problems that can hinder the smooth operation of the such committees, and they must be recognized quickly and acted upon.

The IEC as Physician's Hobby: One of the greatest impediments any IEC is likely to encounter is the physician who comes to view the IEC as his or her "hobby." As we mentioned above, good training for the physician co-chair in how to run a meeting is essential in preventing this. Likewise the other IEC members must have training from the outset to empower them all to say, "Wait a minute, I have something to say."

The IEC as Clinical Discussion Group: The view that an ethical dilemma is really a clinical problem to be solved clinically can reassert itself throughout the life of the committee when physician members try to use the IEC as another a venue for clinical discussions, or view the case as simply another clinical problem to be solved. Since one of the co-chairs will be a physician, and a simple majority of the members may be physicians, this is a constant issue about which all members must be aware.

A structured methodology for case consultation provides the best assurance that the IEC discussion will focus on the ethical issues, with clinical issues a well-defined, and not dominating, part of that discussion. ☐

METHODOLOGY

CASE REVIEW METHODOLOGY

Without a consistent method, the committee can easily develop into a discussion club for a handful of the more vocal or charismatic participants.

A methodology for ethical deliberation, like a methodology for any clinical discipline, seeks to guarantee that all important aspects of a case will be considered and that the quality of a committee's work from patient to patient is consistent. Furthermore, it systematizes and amplifies members' capacity to learn from their experiences.

Without a consistent method, the committee can easily develop into a discussion club for a handful of the more vocal or charismatic participants. Though it may well lead to an interesting and even satisfying discussion, a "seminar" format will not guarantee a consistent and thorough consideration of the issues, nor will it address the necessity for establishing criteria for all cases regardless of the participants' subjective feelings about a particular case or individual patient.

A methodology is also a key factor in the development of the IEC as a **moral community**. By "moral community," we mean a forum of individuals with diverse experiences, professional backgrounds, interests and philosophies of life who offer those who have to make decisions the benefit of the wisdom and advice of their deliberation.

More subtly, and perhaps just as important, the mutual respect members within a moral community have for one another's differences may assist in resolving difficulties just as much as the content of their consultation. By their example as a *community*, they mentor to the general institutional community a new *modus operandi* for conflict resolution quite different from typical clinical relationships; they become identified as a "community within the community" willing to give their time and energy and skill to a type of reflection required in response to ethical dilemmas. A clear, established methodology assists the IEC as a moral community to arrive at clear positions within its diversity, and in so doing, helps create the culture of the IEC.

A methodology is not a recipe for resolution. Nor is it a promise of certainty or facility. It is a way of making a choice, and a mechanism for amplifying the institutional ethics committee's knowledge base. While each IEC will have its own dynamic, and each committee's process will be shaped by the particular history of cases it reviews as it grows, use of a methodology will allow the IEC's culture and knowledge to be cumulative and transmissible.

The following is the Bioethics Consultation Group methodology as it has evolved in the training and support of ethics committees. Our approach is fundamentally different from ones which view ethical consultation as an extension of the clinical skills of individual physicians, or view ethical deliberation as only a matter of facilitating communications among conflicting actors in the clinical setting.

Our approach depends upon the structured deliberation of an ongoing group of individuals representing a variety of disciplines using specific skills and knowledge not commonly found in the training of clinicians. This method guarantees that each case will be treated by the committee in the same organized fashion, and that the IEC will not be thrown off course by exotic and extraneous data. It also assists in adherence to the requirements of justice — the obligation to treat each case equally, and with a uniform procedure.

The BCG methodology is not intended to be a rigid structure to which ethics committee must adhere; rather, its steps have been found to ensure that all necessary information is gathered, appropriately and efficiently structured, and applied to a careful process of analysis in light of specific, concrete choices available to the responsible clinicians, patients and family.

Gatekeeping

For the methodology to be properly applied, the IEC needs to make some careful judgments at the outset about what cases are appropriate for its consideration. Not all the cases referred to the IEC will be appropriate, and the co-chairs should become adept at sorting out what is truly an ethical dilemma and thus appropriate for committee consideration, from what more properly should be referred to other committees or departments of the institution.

The classic example of a situation often mistaken for an ethical problem occurs when a physician devises a treatment plan for a patient, explains that plan to the family, but neglects to tell the primary care nurses the rationale behind it. The primary care nurses may view the level or type of care they're being directed to give as inappropriate given what they know of the patient's situation; to them, it appears to be an ethical problem, but in truth, most of the time it's a communications problem.

However, there's rarely a clear distinction between what is appropriate for IEC consideration, and what is not. Rather there's a continuum from the purely ethical at the one end, to issues such as utilization, interpersonal difficulties, diagnostic fuzziness and communications problems at the other. Unfortunately for the co-chairs, they will rarely encounter a purely ethical dilemma; instead, most ethical dilemmas that are brought before the IEC will be embedded in other problems. For example, in the situation cited above, the physician's rationale for his or her treatment plan may disregard the patient's prior directives concerning withdrawal or withholding of treatment; the family may be conflictive about that prior directive, and what it implies. Thus there may well be an ethical issue — the patient's

autonomy vs. the physician's determination of what's clinically best — tangled into other issues having to do with
communication between the physician and nurses, and the
physician, nurses and family.

Sorting all of this out is an art, and the IEC co-chairs will
need to separate clearly the ethical issues from all the others;
the real skill in gatekeeping is not so much in preventing
cases from coming before the IEC, but in isolating the ethical dilemma from other circumstances once a case does
come to the IEC for review.

"New" IECs tend to dismiss cases when they're not
"pure" ethical dilemmas, which is a mistake since, again,
"pure" ethical dilemmas are rare. Some IECs err the other
way and allow themselves to become embroiled in politics,
or allow themselves to become a forum for airing interpersonal conflicts between physicians, nurses, and others. A
certain balance is called for.

Gatekeeping, in our view, should be a progressive sorting out procedure; as the IEC gathers more and more information about a particular case and gains a deeper understanding of it, they may discover they're not the appropriate forum for discussion, but in all likelihood they will
discover some ethical dimension that is appropriate for
discussion.

If the IEC finally determines that the case in fact has
nothing to do with an ethical dilemma, the committee ought
nonetheless to try to find a way to address the needs of
whoever referred the case in the first place; this may amount
simply to finding some other agency in the institution or
community that is appropriate.

A final word of caution: we strongly recommend against
taking anonymous requests for case review. In many institutions, for a variety of reasons, whether valid or not, nurses

and other healthcare professionals, and even sometimes physicians working as consultants on a case, will bring a case to the IEC co-chairs, saying "You really ought to look at this case, it's a big problem, but don't use my name."

We feel strongly that such cases should not be accepted. Physicians will immediately view the IEC as a policing agency, and they'll be right. If, in considering the request, the co-chairs feel it should be reviewed by the IEC but the person referring it still refuses to allow his or her name to be used, then the co-chairs ought to exercise a bit of creativity at this point, and find a way to get the case before the IEC, most easily by finding someone else to refer the case who *will* use his or her name.

We also feel strongly that there be a specific, formal process in place for referring cases to the IEC. This process should be published, and made available throughout the institution.

There are three advantages to doing so. First, an established, published procedure for case referral tells everyone concerned that the organization takes ethical deliberation seriously enough to make it a formal process. Second, such a formal procedure guarantees protections for those who bring a case to the IEC by demonstrating that the institution does not want to dismiss such problems, but is actively seeking them out. And third, the formal procedure allows the co-chairs to fall back on the process requirements when faced with an anonymous referral. Once a case has been chosen for consideration, the following step-by-step methodology can be applied.

STEP ONE: *The Formal Opening*

The ethical consultation ought to begin with a formal, written opening statement. Read aloud, the statement reminds members of the basic principles of ethical deliberation and assures newcomers that it's permitted, and encouraged, to speak openly about very difficult matters.

Also, the opening statement helps create a space that is quite distinct from the usual hierarchy of the clinical world; here, the committee reminds itself of this difference and that every member of the committee, regardless his or her training or background or place in the institutional reporting structure, has something important to contribute. The opening reiterates and reinforces the basic notion that good ethical deliberation is possible only with the richness of perspectives provided by a diversity of voices, and that such diversity is possible only in an atmosphere of complete confidentiality. Finally, the opening reminds everyone that the committee's ultimate purpose is the welfare of the patient.

We believe the opening should be formal. We've seen committees in which a chairperson will make a few casual opening remarks, but these remarks tend to reflect whatever she or he is thinking about at the moment. The ritual should reiterate the same fundamental principles each time.

The actual introductory statement should be the creation of the particular committee. The formulation of this statement serves as a "constituting document" for the early period of the IEC's development, and its repetition, in a sense, reconstitutes the IEC with each case review meeting. (Please see Figure #2, page 57.)

While each IEC will write its own opening statement, that statement will probably touch on certain key elements:

(1) a presumption of good will of all participants in the deliberation;

(2) the necessity for confidentiality;

(3) the principle of patient-centered decision-making;

(4) the collegial relationship of those on the IEC;

(5) a clear welcome for family members;

(6) an acknowledgement of the special role of the patient's primary caregivers;

(7) and a clear understanding that the IEC's role is to make recommendations, not decisions.

Presumption of Good Will: The statement should assert that the IEC is a mutually supportive community gathered in **good will**. If there are members or guests who have discernible motives that could be considered prejudicial to the case, they ought to be identified. Examples of prejudicial factors are a close personal relationship with the patient, a financial relationship that might be affected by any recommendation of the IEC, or an overriding categorical stand toward a certain genre of patient (e.g., "I simply cannot work with a drug abusing parent"). Though such factors won't necessarily preclude an individual from IEC deliberations, they ought to be expressed and evaluated.

In this, as at many points in the deliberative process, truth telling and plain speaking are essential. There should be no ideas or felt realities that are "not acceptable" for discussion, and the co-chairs should facilitate discussion and see to it that all voices are heard. Holding back with certain ideas for fear of being judged "unethical" is of no help to the committee, the patient, or the involved healthcare team, since these suppressed ideas may be expressed covertly, usually in some less than constructive way.

Despite the opening statement's call for a presumption of good will, longstanding institutional "traditions" or established ways in which staff relate to one another can make such a presumption difficult for some. In particular, nurses in some institutions have a hard time accepting the notion they can speak freely in front of physicians without later ramifications; too often, they see themselves as a pair of hands simply carrying out orders, rather than as separate moral agents with a need to think through what they're doing, and why. Again, the opening serves to reinforce for everyone present how important it is that *all* members speak out, and that they can do so safely. Thus the next principle, the principle of **confidentiality**, can't be overemphasized.

Confidentiality: The confidence of all committee members in the inviolability of confidentiality makes disclosure and discussion of all ideas possible; confidentiality is thus basic to the committee's functioning. It is also a basic patient right.

Since hospital standards of confidentiality vary widely in practice, the opening statement should reinforce this principle. IEC members need to hear again and again that the principle of confidentiality is absolute, however lax hospital standards of confidentiality may be outside the committee deliberations. The process of ethical deliberation cannot proceed without the clear understanding that the door of the room is firmly closed and no names will ever be attached to any case discussed outside the room. And, most importantly, all opinions expressed in the room will be confidential and never discussed in any other capacity or any other venue.

Patient-Centered Decision-Making: The opening statement ought to express a commitment to patient- centered decision-making. This means that the primary focus is on the patient. While other factors will be given serious consideration in the discourse, the IEC will have a clear bias for the patient's best interests.

Collegial Relationships: At many times in the hospital or other clinical setting, physician/non-physician relationships are structured by the need for a clear hierarchical decision-making process. The process of ethics case review is a different arena, however, in which the wisdom of the nurse, of the community members, the social worker, the administrator and the physician are all of equal importance. Each member will be asked to reflect on the case and must be honored and respected without regard to his or her place in the clinical hierarchy. Building a **moral community** makes this an essential part of the work.

Welcome to Families: When patients or their families attend the consultation meeting, they should be welcomed. We advocate the fullest family participation in this process, if the family so chooses. But the judgment of whether the family attends the entire meeting, a portion, or whether the providers meet with the family separately prior to or after the committee's deliberations, is a matter determined primarily by the maturity of the committee.

Committees mature at different rates, but any committee that is still experimenting with the process may not be comfortable if a patient's family is present. A more mature committee whose members trust one another and in which the ground rules of open discussion and plain speaking have been habitualized, may be much more comfortable.

Two things should be stressed when families attend: first, the family is *not* at a tribunal, and they will not be judged by the committee; second, kinship does not mean ownership of the patient. While family input is an *imperative* voice for the committee to hear, it is *not* an absolute voice. Most families are reassured and heartened by sincere efforts to consider the case of their family member and are pleased the IEC has given them this extra time.

Patient's Primary Caregivers: In a parallel fashion, the IEC should acknowledge the special place at the table of the **patient's primary caregivers.** These physicians, nurses, social workers and other clinicians should understand that their relationship and advocacy will be honored, that their opinions and responses will be the heart of the discussion, and that nothing is unsafe to say at the meeting.

primary caregivers

Recommendation, Not A Decision: Finally, the goal of the meeting is to make a clear and coherent recommendation to the attending physician or whoever requested the consultation, and to offer a discourse that will be helpful in the process of his or her final clinical decision. A **recommendation and not a decision** is the goal of the meeting.

recommendation, not a decision

At the outset, clear limits on the time allowed for the discussion and recommendation should be set, typically an hour to an hour-and-a-half.

STEP TWO: *Identify the Presenter*

Having read the formal opening, the next step in the committee process is to identify the presenter. Any member of the healthcare team may bring a case to the committee, as can the patient or family. In any case, the attending physician should be present, particularly if the primary care nurse or other non-physician caregiver has brought the case to the committee; likewise, if the primary physician has brought the case, then other relevant caregivers should attend.

Sometimes, the issues will present primarily as a physician/nurse conflict, or a breakdown in communication between the physician and nurses, and the case should be addressed as such. Again, the committee co-chairs must become skilled gatekeepers here to separate truly ethical issues from the other issues such as staff conflicts.

STEP THREE: *Identify the Problem*

The co-chair of the IEC should next ask the presenter for an initial problem statement. The IEC should pay close attention to the language used here, for this language will determine the moral scope of the discussion. How is the question framed? What is it that is disturbing the presenter? What is the presenter's description of the ethical dilemma?

Words such as "kill" or "starve," for example, should be red flags. The committee needs to take note of the loaded language used in the case of a presenter who, for example, says the issue is whether or not to put in a feeding tube or to let a patient "starve," and in such a case try to understand what's bothering the presenter, and what the presenter is trying to express.

The co-chairs can help in this process by focusing the question and making sure the most pertinent questions are asked; in the case of the use or withdrawal of a feeding tube, for example, the real questions may well be: What is the patient's wish? Can this be ascertained? Did the patient leave a durable power of attorney? Who can speak for the patient?

The statement of the problem may well change as the process of ethical deliberation moves forward, but the initial statement will nonetheless tell the IEC much about the values and belief structures that underlie the intellectual issues at stake.

STEP FOUR: Information Gathering

A comprehensive and detailed matrix (please see Figure #3, page 59) as a way to enter the discussion about a particular case, will organize and categorize all the information available to the ethics committee in a systematic and comprehensive fashion. As mentioned above, this establishes that each case will be treated by the committee in the same organized fashion and assists in adherence to the requirements of justice.

There are several broad categories of information the IEC will need to gather: medical information, information about patient preferences, the social location of each patient, social and economic factors, and staff input. It's not necessary to supply information for all the parts of the matrix, however. Some types of information asked for on the matrix may not be applicable to the particular case in question; the matrix is simply a tool to help the IEC cover all the material that will be necessary for a thorough discussion of each particular case. Categories of information include:

I. Medical: This section begins with a concise medical history: the diagnosis and prognosis and the history and result of each medical intervention. Questions to ask include:

- **What was expected of each medical intervention?**
- **What is the long term expectation of care?**

In lay terms, the IEC needs to know:

- **What went wrong?**
- **What has the healthcare team done?**
- **What do they think will happen?**

Each medical term will need to be carefully explained in the most direct language possible, not only for the community members present, but for healthcare practitioners not familiar with the particular medical specialty under discussion.

In cases in which withdrawing or withholding treatment is the issue, the single most important question may be the one that is hardest to ask, and to answer:

- **Is the patient dying?**

This issue, often avoided in clinical medicine, must be faced head-on by the IEC. Where is the patient in her or his life trajectory? Is the patient at an end stage event in a terminal disease? At a crisis in a chronic, debilitating but essentially stable state? Will the medical effort be "futile?"

Incidentally, the determination of futility is a medical question, apart from the moral import of the question, and in light of the great and continuing debate over the use of the term "futility" in the current medical literature, we suggest great specificity at this point: **futility** as we use the term refers to treatments that will not stop the inevitability of death, or to treatments that will not affect the specific condition, or to treatments that are physiologically unsound.

By asking whether intervention will be futile, we're asking: Will the proposed intervention affect a cure, or a solution to the underlying cause of disease? Will the patient die in any case, and will the course of his or her disease be unaffected by the care?

Quality of life is not an issue here; intervention is not futile if it results in a diminished quality of life. There are words that can describe an effort of this sort; such a treatment might be called "not therapeutic," or "non-efficacious" or "burdensome" in a way that is disproportionate to the benefits, but it is not necessarily futile. Futility can only be judged in light of specific goals.

Also relevant to the discussion about the patient's medical condition is research about the disease, the reports from other consulting physicians, lab results, and, most importantly, the **outcome statistics** for prospective treatments.

II. Patient Preferences:
This is central to the entire IEC deliberation: **What does the patient want?** This is a complex question. The following questions may help to sort out the necessary information:

futility

quality of life

*What does the
patient want?*

- **What does the patient say?**
- **What did the patient write if the patient
  is unconscious?**
- **What did the patient say or write to a legal
  surrogate if the patient lives in a state with
  a DPA for healthcare?**
- **What did the guardian know of the patient's
  desires if guardianship is legally
  established?**

Certainly, the **conscious** patient must be asked what she or he wants, even if the practitioner is concerned that the patient will not fully understand, that his or her judgment is clouded by the condition of the illness, or that the patient will be overwhelmed by the implications of the questions being asked.

The IEC should be clear here about the distinction between a patient's **competency**, a legal term, and **capacity**, a medical judgment (please see Ethical Theory, page 18, for more on this). A conscious patient may legally be competent, but his or her capacity to understand may nonetheless be in question. On the other hand, the IEC also needs to understand that even when a conscious patient may no longer be able to make decisions in other areas of his or her life, the capacity to make decisions about his or her body, and to say "Touch me" or "Don't touch me," may remain intact.

III. Family Systems There are a variety of cases in which the IEC won't be able to ascertain the patient's desires, however. Examples include:

(1) **Pediatric and neonatology patients** — Infants are by

competency
vs. capacity

family systems

definition incapable of autonomous decision-making; decision-makers are always making **best interests judgments** on their behalf. The IEC must consider family input at this point: in most cases, we assume the family makes decisions in the best interests of the patient, unless evidence points to the contrary. Great care is advisable when confronted with the tragedy of a dysfunctional family, however. The IEC's role is definitely not to act as court, diagnostician or therapist for such a family, but rather to refer the matter to appropriate social services. At the same time, the IEC should be cognizant of issues of provider bias in making assumptions about whether or not a family "loves" a patient enough.

As for the decision-making capacity of older children, under the law, they are not *competent*. However, as children develop, especially in adolescence, they will demonstrate an increasing *capacity* to make decisions for themselves and what they want done to their bodies. The older child and adolescent, when conscious, should be involved in decisions about his or her care.

(2) Patients in a persistent vegetative state: While these patients will never again be able to state a preference, they almost always have a history of competent adulthood. If there is no prior *written* or *verbal statement* of wishes, the IEC should seek other sources for insights into what the patient would have wanted. Here, the IEC seeks first to help the family to recall what the patient may have said regarding care decisions and to assist them in separating their own preferences from the patient's desires. It may be helpful for the IEC to ask:

- **Who are the real decision-makers in this family?**
- **What is the meaning of this tragedy for them?**

(While it is the IEC's "work" to be here, it is always, to the family, singularly, *their* tragedy. It will be remembered as a "case" or a "story" by the practitioners, but it will be the daily lived reality for the family. They will take it home, and know it in a way the IEC members cannot. The IEC should be sensitive to this, and maintain the family's dignity and its own humility in the face of this truth.)

- **Who will speak for the family? Is this the decision-maker? The only one who speaks English (or "science")? The IEC must be careful to hear the other voices in the family system.**
- **Who will care for the patient?**
- **Who has cared for the patient?**
- **Who lives with whom?**
- **Is the very quiet woman in the back of the room the one who will love the child — or the enfeebled older adult — the most?**

The IEC *can* assume, in most cases, that the family knows the patient's wishes because the family members simply know and love the patient better than anyone else. But the practitioners are also realists who live in a world where this is sometimes not the case. The IEC must be very cautious when making assumptions about the love a family feels for a patient based on such limited information as frequency of visits, however.

Sometimes, children of aging parents will want a level of care that is not medically reasonable, because it is experienced as reparations for loving care given to them as children. Sometimes, a distant child who rarely visited the

parent will view withdrawal of treatment as abandonment,
for which he or she feels guilty. Also, everyone involved
should understand that children and vulnerable adults are
not the *property* of their families.

When the IEC explores the case with families, it can
make it safe for the family candidly to describe their limits,
the picture of the family life that they envision, and what
they can expect in the way of realistic support.

IV. Community Involvement: The idea of the "family"
needs to be defined broadly; in some cases, we need to look
beyond blood ties or legal bonds such as marriage. We also
need to consider cultural differences in terms of family ties;
different cultures can have different family dynamics, and
the IEC needs to consider these as well.

The social location of each patient is a key part of
understanding the dilemma. In many cases (for example,
the adult with an AIDS diagnosis who is estranged from his
or her family), the community and not the family is the
relevant social support system. It is common that a religious
community (a church, congregation or synagogue) will be
the "community of meaning" that is most central to the
patient. However, it may also be the union, a political club,
friends at work, the neighborhood, etc.

The IEC shouldn't overlook the critical importance of
any social or "lifestyle enclaves" in the patient's life; it's
helpful for committee members to remember that they'll
see the patient in one dramatic moment of her or his life.
Considering who the person is in his or her community,
why that person lives in a particular way, and to whom that
person is responsible are questions which may be helpful in
case review.

community
involvement

V. Social and Economic Factors: There is usually a strong taboo against airing questions of cost during a case review. This attitude is understandable, but unrealistic in the context of the economic realities that face any patient, family or clinician.

We know from our own experience at the bedside that virtually all decisions about the withdrawal of treatment evoke the question "Is all this worth it?", and that practitioners mean this, at least in part, in the economic sense.

As all practitioners come face to face with the realities of scarcity, the tension around allocation of resources will increase. The question can mean not only "Can this family afford the cost of the care?", but "Can we as an institution afford this care?" Many ethics committees refuse to discuss this openly. Instead, this discussion happens covertly, at the bedside, at the nurse's station, in the doctor's lounge. Practitioners believe so strongly in the principle that every single human life is of infinite value that it is painful to acknowledge that the practitioner operates in institutions where resource constraints are real. The IEC needs to be open about the question: **who will pay and what is the real cost?**

It's helpful to know the cost in both economic and social terms. What is the insurance situation? (This will impact heavily on the family's concerns.) What are the limits of long-term coverage? What are the discharge plans? What is the impact of the case on the unit? How are staffing patterns affected? Is the hospital on diversion, desperate for any space it can get, or is it eager to fill beds? Who staffs this patient, the registry or the most highly trained nurse? How are the other patients affected by this case and by this family?

Discussing these issues openly gets back to one of the

fundamental principles of committee deliberation, the **presumption of good will** and the clear understanding by all that no subject is taboo, and that all topics are suitable for discussion.

Finally, the IEC may want to consider the social implications of any case. The committee's role is not to discuss strategies for a response to the public, but it should reflect on possible social implications of any recommendation, and be prepared, if the case at hand somehow becomes a public issue, to explain to the community as a whole the ethical decision-making process that led to a recommendation.

The presence of community members on the committee is enormously valuable when discussing the social implications of any case since they are often most aware of the concerns of a community; they can bring a touch of "reality" into the sometimes rarified atmosphere of individual case deliberation.

VI. Staff Input: At this point in the process, each appropriate staff member involved in the case (the physician, house officer, nurse, social worker, technicians and others) should each have a chance to express his or her ethical opinions about the case and dilemma under review. Here, the IEC is looking for the kind of *subjective* moral reflections that were excluded in previous steps of the process.

The IEC may request the caregivers' assessments of all the facts: what is said in rounds, in candid discussion among the primary care staff. And here it's wise to reiterate the principle of confidentiality. Each staff member must be assured that no statement will place him or her in personal jeopardy. Further, all related staff opinions are welcome.

Often, each particular nursing shift will have unique

and important views of the patient and family which will help in the deliberation; perhaps the family only visits on the p.m. shift, for example, so that shift may have special insights to offer the committee. It is imperative that all involved staff be included.

VII. Daily Life: As noted above, this information gathering matrix has no place on it for "quality of life" determinations. Despite the very popular use of this notion in the ethics literature, it is difficult to imagine how a group of healthcare professionals, predominantly white and able-bodied, highly educated, and by definition high achieving and successful, could accurately judge another's "quality of life" across racial, cultural, ethnic, and class lines. It is particularly difficult for the able-bodied to assess the life experience of the differently abled person, even when this assessment isn't compounded by the enormous cultural confusion about what a "good life" is. Ultimately, only the patient can make this determination; if the patient is comatose and can't express his or her views on the matter, then such issues should not arise. Our opining that the life of another is or is not of good quality usually reflects our own value systems projected onto the patient.

What the IEC *can* determine, however, is the daily life of the person as patient in the institution's care. The IEC can ask: What does this person do at 7 a.m., at 8 a.m., at 9, 10, 11 and so on throughout the day? The IEC can ask the primary care nurses, who sit by the bedside and closely observe, what is actually done to the patient, and how does the patient react to procedures as they're performed? Does the day begin with chest PT and suction, followed by lab draws? Is it a series of painful interventions, one after the other, or are there long hours when the patient seems to be

daily life

quality of life

Our opining that the life of another is or is not of good quality usually reflects our own value systems projected onto the patient.

having a comfortable and restful time? In the case of the comatose or the very young who cannot verbalize their experience, such a description will be enormously valuable.

In all cases, an hour-by-hour description can give the committee a clear picture of the patient's experience, and only as shown on the outside, not, of course, as the person may experience it himself or herself. Often, family members and even physicians or residents may only see the patient for a rather brief period, and can easily come in at a "high" or "low" moment in the treatment course. A line graphing the pleasure and pain expressed, or observed, will enable the IEC to "see" as the bedside nurse can see this patient.

This picture is crucial; this sort of visual account can help the IEC members understand why, for example, a patient on a ventilator wants the treatment discontinued. Most likely no committee member has ever been a ventilated patient in the ICU or experienced the suctions, medications, and percussive therapies that are routine. For IEC members, the pain and disorientation a patient feels through it all is likely an abstraction. But hearing from a primary caregiver about a patient's series of painful interventions one after another with only brief periods of rest makes the patient's experience much more concrete and accessible.

(Please note, all the categories listed above can be gathered by the co-chairs prior to the actual meeting; copies of the matrix with relevant categories filled in can be distributed at the meeting. However, these items still should be reviewed by the entire committee in the meeting.)

VIII. The Ideal Picture: We strongly recommend at the end of the information-gathering process that the members of the IEC individually answer the question: What is your ideal picture? and: Can you really offer this to the patient?

There may be no room for wish fulfillment at the decision-making level, but here the question should be asked, since it allows for the paternalistic and basically good-hearted visions of the providers to be made overt, and for the healthcare team to gauge how far from possibility their desires really are. Once voiced, the yearning for an orderly world and for control can be noted, reflected upon, and when necessary, put aside.

the "howevers"

IX. The "Howevers": This is also the time for the IEC members to ask if there's any information that has been missed, a final review to assure thoroughness. Is there an overpowering or outstanding legal consideration here? Is there a court case pending that is relevant? The IEC might also want to ask here if there's a public relations issue to be considered, is the press involved, or is the family threatening to sue? All these small elements can make a significant difference, and they may not be captured by the categories in the matrix.

STEP FIVE: *Outcomes*

The next step in the method narrows the wide range of ideas and information into two or more decision options, and one of the most creative and useful things the IEC can do at this point is to point out that there may be third and fourth options. When confronted with ethical dilemmas, there's a tendency toward a bipolar structure of thought: I can do *this* or I can do *that*.

But there may be courses of action that no one has thought of, and the IEC should help everyone involved explore these other possibilities and break free from the bipolar way of thinking. This is where you want expansive thinking, where you want people to be creative about options and think broadly.

The IEC will eventually choose options that are actual treatment plans, and see them as possible roads to follow. Since each action option will have consequence, some beneficial, some burdensome, upon the various actors identified by the IEC — not just on the patient, but on the family, the healthcare team and even society — the committee needs to assess these benefits and burdens and follow each treatment plan for some probable distance into the future. At this juncture, the IEC should not attach values to the outcomes, but simply discuss what the results are likely to be, and the effects on the various actors.

The options can be general in scope. Later, when the IEC works toward consensus, it may make more refined recommendations. At this point, it's sufficient to narrow the choice to the most basic options, for example, "full treatment" versus "comfort measures only."

The IEC then asks what will be the benefits and the burdens of each course on each actor, carefully and systematically following the form (please see Figure #4, page 60) for each possible option and for each person involved.

Throughout the information gathering and benefit-and-burden analysis phase of the process, the IEC may began to identify issues and options as exemplifying different ethical principles such as **autonomy, justice, beneficence, staff integrity** and so on (please refer to Ethical Theory). Committee members will begin to see the theoretical grounding beyond the outcomes, and to reflect on the values that underlie the choices that must be made in each particular case. Over time, this will contribute to the committee's development as a moral community, and to the richness of its deliberations.

STEP SIX: *Deliberation*

When the options, with benefits and burdens, have been charted, the committee is ready to rank values (please see Figure #5, page 61) and discern which of the many competing values each will rank most highly, for example a patient's autonomy versus the physician's desire to do what he or she deems clinically most effective.

There will be many ways to assess the rightness of an option, to assess **what is the right act, and what makes it right.** Some will decide based on the principle of **consequentialism/utilitarianism** (please refer to Ethical Theory for more on this); looking at the outcome graph, they'll choose that act which will create the greatest happiness or greatest "good" for the greatest number involved in the case. Some may use a **duty-based** (deontological) approach, looking at the motives behind an action. Still others may work at finding a rule or deriving a rule from this or previous cases that smooth the path to a decision (casuistry), rather than beginning with principles to apply to the case. And still others will look at the case and find their decisions based on an allegiance to one or more of the classic principles of bioethics — **beneficence, non-maleficence, justice and autonomy.** Some will follow Aristotle and ask not "What should I do?" but rather "Who should I be?" and base their decision on how they see their virtues, and what is a virtuous way to act, the **virtue-based** approach.

Going around the table, each person should answer the

question: **Which option did you choose and why did you choose it?** At this time, the co-chairs will want to note if there is a consensus, although this in no way constitutes a vote. The IEC will offer a consensus recommendation if there is a clear majority in favor of one option. If the committee is divided and no consensus emerges, the recommendation ought to reflect this fact.

Finally, though most cases can be discussed to resolution in one meeting, some decisions take more than one session, and if the case warrants, the IEC may meet again.

STEP SEVEN: *Legal Issues*

Legal considerations should be discussed only at the end of the process; ethical discourse should always come prior to any discussion of legal implications (please refer to Legal Issues for more on this).

Many healthcare providers have a strong fear that the law will act in a way that will constrain essential moral values — "I'd like to do this, but my hands are tied." In fact, the law is only beginning to address the problems inherent in many of the finely nuanced decisions the IEC will give advice about, and in many, many cases, there is as yet no national or even state consensus on practice, thus the provider's fears of legal constraint are usually unfounded.

Law, like medicine, is subject to a wide variety of interpretations. Lawyers, like physicians and nurses, can and will disagree on the "diagnosis" or assessment of the situation and the best remedy. It is important to remember that **good medicine leads to good ethics and this directs good law.** Legal consensus will emerge as more cases are adjudi-

...the provider's fears of legal constraint are usually unfounded.

cated. Meanwhile, each institution will have legal counsel who can advise on the specifics of the law as it will affect the life of the particular institution and the particular patient. Once a decision for a recommendation has been reached, legal counsel can discuss with the group what law may affect this case. We do believe that ethics committees need to know the precedential cases in the bioethics literature. (Please refer to Getting Started and Legal Issues for more on the use of legal counsel as consultants or IEC members.)

STEP EIGHT: *Recording*

There are three distinct layers of reporting that are necessary (please refer to Getting Started for more on this). These are: (1) a brief, general summary of the proceedings, usually simply frequency reports, for whatever body the IEC reports to, be it the Medical Staff Executive Committee or the administration; (2) a detailed report to the person bringing the case to the committee; and (3) a narrative, structured account of the case for the committee's own files and education. The attached form (please see Figure #6, page 62) is intended to go on the chart *if the MD chooses.* In any case, it is filed as a specific record of the decision.

The IEC should also note who will follow up, if further discussion is necessary, or if more data are needed. One of the tasks of the committee is to assure that all referrals are followed up by a designated individual. By the next committee meeting, a report about the case should be submitted to the group. The treating physician and primary care nurse need to be clear on what happened at the committee level and the committee needs to know if more is expected of it.

The IEC's "Product":

A final consideration regarding the methodology is the IEC's "product." What is it, exactly, that the IEC provides? The product of the IEC's deliberations is not, of course, a decision about what will happen to the patient or what the patient will do; only the patient, the patient's family, and the patient's physicians can decide that.

Rather, the IEC's product, in the broadest sense, is the richest possible moral reflection around an ethical dilemma. In a narrower sense, the IEC will try to arrive at a consensus about a specific *recommendation* for the patient, the patient's physician, and the family.

Thus the IEC, in the process of deliberation, is deciding not what the physician or patient or family will do, but rather it is deciding what *it* will recommend. This isn't to say that the IEC will always come up with a consensus recommendation. There will be times when the complexity of issues and the diversity of perceptions involved make a consensus unlikely; in that case it is the richness of the IEC's deliberations that the IEC will ultimately provide. ☐

Figure #1 The Process: Methodology for Case Review

---

1. THE RITUAL OPENING: CREATION OF TIME AND SPACE
   FOR REFLECTION:

   - Presume Good Will
   - Confidentiality is Primary
   - Patient Centered Decision-making
   - Collegial Relationship is Essential
   - Family Input is Valued, Welcomed and Invited
   - Patient's Primary Caregivers are Valued and Welcomed
   - Recommendation and not Decision is the Goal

2. IDENTIFY THE PRESENTER

3. IDENTIFY PRESENTING PROBLEM

4. INFORMATION GATHERING:

   - Medical Information
   - Family System
   - Staff Input
   - Daily Life
   - Patient Preferences
   - Community Involvement
   - Social/Economic Considerations
   - The Ideal Picture
   - Is There More To Say?

5. CHART BENEFITS AND BURDENS

6. RANK VALUES

7. COMING TO A CONSENSUS

8. SUMMATION

Figure #2   Sample Opening

PREAMBLE TO CASE REVIEW

1. Meeting at the request of _________________.
To discuss:_________________________________.

2. Case of _________________________________.

Before we introduce ourselves, it is important that we remember that everyone comes with the patient's best interest at heart and with a deep respect for patient confidentiality.

3. Introductions of the committee members and of those invited due to their involvement in the case or invited as outside consultants. Introductions here include a brief statement of position in the institution or relation to the patient. Note: Indicate before these introductions if family members are present and introduce them.

4. If family members are not present, determine if they have been informed of the review.

It is important to understand that the Ethics Committee does not sit in judgement, and does not make decisions for physicians, patients and families.

The purpose of the Ethics Committee is to provide an open forum to discuss differing opinions in an open and nonjudgmental way; to assure through this process that the highest level of decision making is accomplished. All input is desired. We all respect the right of others to have different opinions and different values.

Ethics Committee deliberations are moved out of the strictly medical areas and into the realm of process, values and decision making.

The Ethics Committee defines an ethical issue as a conflict of values. Through this process we will attempt to identify the relevant values, the conflicts around these values, and the options available to the patient, patient's family and the physician.

The committee process attempts to achieve a consensus which will permit resolution of the conflict. A written summary of the Ethics Committee consultation and recommendation will be given to the primary physician and will be placed in the patient's medical record.

5. The process of ethical consultation includes a medical summary, psychosocial input, nursing input, family input — if present — and other.

6. We'll list actual options possible and both positive and negative values/outcomes achieved for patient/family/staff, and identify where any conflicts lie.

7. We'll attempt to achieve consensus on an acceptable option, with the understanding that the success of our discussion does not depend on consensus, which may not always be possible, or necessarily desirable. Rather, success will depend on the richness of perspectives provided.

8. The process is important in that it is to be an open forum where conflicting options may be aired.

9. The results of the consultation are advisory and the primary decision makers remain the patient, physician and the family.

________________________ will now present the case.

Figure #3   Information Gathering: a Worksheet

Medical Information

Patient Preferences

Family System

Community Involvement

Staff Input

Social/Economic Considerations

Daily Life

The Ideal Picture

Is there more to say? Are there issues that make this case distinctive?

Figure #4   Charting Benefits and Burdens

Major Actors	Benefits	Burdens
Option One — 1. 2. 3. 4.		
Option Two — 1. 2. 3. 4.		
*Option Three** — 1. 2. 3. 4.		

**Note: there is no limit on the number of options.*

COMING TO CONSENSUS: STATING VALUES AND PRINCIPLES

GENERAL VALUES RE: QUESTION

SPECIFIC VALUES RE: QUESTION WITH THIS *PATIENT*

COMING TO CONSENSUS: REFLECTING ON VALUES

COURSE OF ACTION: MOTIVATING VALUE:

OPTION ONE

OPTION TWO

OPTION THREE

RANKING OPTIONS:

RATIONALE

LEGAL CONSIDERATIONS:

RELEVANT CASE LAW OR PRECEDENT

Figure #6   Summation

SUMMATION OF THE CONSULTATIVE PROCESS

Name of attending M.D.________________MR#________________Pt.
Patients Name____

Date________________
Facility________________

BRIEF CASE SUMMARY:

ETHICAL ISSUE(S):

RECOMMENDATION:

IMPLEMENTATION:

PLANS FOR FOLLOW-UP/TIME SCHEDULE:

THANK YOU FOR THE OPPORTUNITY TO CONSIDER THIS CASE

ETHICAL THEORY

Ethics And Morality Defined

I n most situations, the answers to the fundamental question of what is best or right are so clear or simple that we're not even aware of the process that leads to them. However, in the healthcare setting in particular, where lives can hang in the balance and providers, patients and family members may all have very individual perspectives on difficult issues, easy answers about what is best or right are not always forthcoming.

The IEC exists precisely because well meaning men and women — healthcare professionals, patients and their families — *can* differ, and differ widely, on what is best or right. They have different values and when these values come into conflict, it is the goal of the IEC to provide a forum for *all* perspectives to be heard and openly discussed. Keep in mind that the IEC is just that, an *ethics* committee; it's not a *morals* committee. To understand the IEC's fundamental purpose and role in providing a forum for differing and perhaps conflicting values and perspectives, it's important to understand at the outset the clear distinction between **morality** and **ethics**.

Morality:

Morality has to do with one's *belief* about what is the right or best thing to do. These can include religious traditions, lessons learned in families about right and wrong, professional codes, and so on.

Two qualities characterize all moral traditions: (1) Within a given tradition, there is a *consensus* of values about what is right or wrong, a unifying code of behavior; and (2) there's an authority or "translator" to which one can turn for answers about what is the right thing to do in a particular case. Priests, rabbis, and professional codes are examples of "authorities" that might be consulted for a translation of what the tradition would recommend in a particular case. So, for example, the nurse might look to the American Nursing Association (ANA) Code of Ethics, the physician to the Hippocratic Oath or the American Medical Association (AMA) Code of Ethics, and the Orthodox Jewish patient to the rabbi or relevant text. These "authorities" can point in a specific direction, and at least give a general sense of what the tradition (i.e., the professional code or religion) would say to do, if not a clear answer. There may be considerable and even ongoing debate within a specific tradition about what is good or right, of course, but often out of that debate comes broad consensus on basic issues.

The problem in a pluralistic, highly diverse society such as ours is that there are many different traditions with distinct and, at times, conflicting values. If we leave things at the level of morality and if each of us simply appeals to his or her own moral traditions to gain insight into what to do, we would never move forward as a society; each moral tradition would have its own values and "speak" its own "language." There would be no common ground or basis for communication and action, which is where the process of ethics comes in.

Ethics:

Ethics is a *process* of reflection that aims to transcend the diversity of moral traditions when responding to value conflicts about what is right and what is wrong. It's clearly distinguished from morality — where there's consensus — precisely because it takes as its starting point a *conflict* of values. In fact, one definition of an ethical dilemma is a situation in which there is a conflict of values, where there's no clear consensus about what's right or wrong, and no single, generally acceptable code of behavior everyone can turn to for insight and guidance.

Because we live in a diverse society, the process of ethics is the best hope we have for coming together as a community to confront difficult questions about values. The purpose of the IEC is to facilitate that process, transcending differences of values to find a common ground or language as a basis for an action decision. ☐

Ethical Schools Of Thought

Ethics begins by asking "what is a good or right act and what makes it so?" Within the Western tradition, there are several schools of ethical thought. Three of the most prominent approaches to the basic questions of ethics are: (1) **consequentialism/utilitarianism;** (2) **deontology**; and (3) the **virtue** or **character-based** approach. Each of us, whether consciously or not, applies the principles of these three schools in our own ethical thinking when trying to decide what is best in a given situation; we'll wonder what the consequences of an act will be (consequentialism); we may examine our own motives for wanting to act a certain way (deontology); and we may well wonder what type of person a given decision will reveal us to be (virtue-based).

Few of us apply the principles of any one of these schools exclusively. Rather, each of us most likely applies all three to a given problem, though we may lean toward one approach over the other two, often depending on the particular circumstances as well as our own training and experience.

IEC members need be familiar with these three schools of thought *not* to categorize their own thinking into a specific school, nor to categorize the thinking of others into schools, but instead to have a broader base from which to consider the questions raised by conflicting values. The goal is not to limit yourself to any one school of thought, but rather to take insights from all three. Familiarity with and appreciation of all three schools of thought will enable you to understand the views of others, and how and why they may differ from yours. The overall result is a richer, more finely nuanced deliberation.

IEC members should avoid appealing to the different schools of thought and applying their associated principles as a sort of "cookbook" for easy ethical decision-making.

The goal is not to limit yourself to any one school of thought, but rather to take insights from all three.

Each ethical dilemma that comes before you will be complex and difficult and *all* perspectives must be brought into the discussion about the question.

In a sense, the product of the IEC is a *full* discussion by well-intentioned and well-trained men and women who know what questions to ask, and who are prepared to discuss the question from a variety of perspectives. Out of that discussion will come a *recommendation* by the IEC to the involved parties (the IEC does not make decisions for caregivers, patient or family, but rather recommendations based on a thorough consideration of a specific case.)

Thus, to ensure the appropriate functioning of the IEC, members should be encouraged to express their opinions fully, even if doing so threatens to break an emerging consensus in the group. In fact, if consensus is reached too readily, someone in the group might assume the role of "devil's advocate" to ensure that all perspectives have been considered. Familiarity with different ethical schools of thought will facilitate this important intervention.

Consequentialism/Utilitarianism:

As the name suggests, "consequentialism" is concerned with consequences. The question being asked is: What's going to happen if I do *this*? What will be the outcome of this action, behavior or policy? When considering aggressive treatment versus withholding treatment in the case of a premature and severely brain damaged newborn, for example, a consequentialist perspective will ask what either option will do to the patient, the family, and society as a whole. Consequentialists begin with these questions because their objective is to maximize good consequences and minimize bad ones. In general, consequentialism defines a good act as one which, on balance, produces more good consequences than bad ones. (Utilitarianism is the best-known subspecies of consequentialism; utilitarians define "good" outcomes in terms of their overall utility. Questions about motive or obligation are less important.)

The consequentialist approach is widely used in the worlds of public policy and clinical decision-making. When decisions are based on a cost/benefit analysis or on the desire to produce the greatest good for the greatest number, they are influenced by the consequentialist perspective.

There are a number of problems with the consequentialist way of thinking, however. First, it still begs the question of what are good consequences and whose perspective should decide? There may well be significant disagreements among physicians, nurses, patient and family over what would be a good consequence for a particular patient, for example; from one perspective, withdrawal of treatment might result in good consequences, while from a quite different perspective, aggressive treatment might produce the most good.

A more fundamental problem with consequentialism concerns its application at the policy level. Because the focus of consequentialism is on the aggregate balance of good and bad consequences, individuals can be sacrificed for the greater good. This is especially the case when the maxim of "the greatest good for the greatest number" is taken as the guiding principle.

Despite these shortcomings, consequentialism in its various forms does provide a respectable starting point in evaluating the question, "What is the best thing to do in this particular circumstance?"

Deontology:

While consequentialism addresses the question of what is a good act and what makes it good with its emphasis on outcomes and consequences, the theory of **deontology** says that what's *really* important in judging whether an action is good or not is what motives underlie that action. What did the actor *intend*? What did the actor *mean* to accomplish? However, this doesn't mean that one's personal desires are paramount. Indeed, deontological theory emphasizes **duty** and **obligation** as transcending law and personal need.

The meaning of "deontology" is "science of duty." Deontology takes the consistent view that the fundamental organizing principle of ethics is **duty**. The meaning of duty cannot be separated from the meaning of **obligation**; essentially, we focus on what ought to be done, and what we're responsible for. Our ability to understand our duty makes us fully human, and fully moral. When considering the case of the brain damaged newborn, the deontological perspective will ask what duties do we have to this patient, what do we *owe* this human being, regardless of the patient's medical condition.

Using duty as a motive for action is usually regarded as unconditional, meaning that it's not subjected to situations or personalities. Duty *requires* ethical action; we perform an action without looking at a balance sheet of costs and benefits to ourselves, based on the outcomes. This notion of the importance of motive derives from Immanuel Kant, who argued that we have a duty to act self-consciously and intentionally in accordance with our faculty of reason.

All of this presupposes that persons have absolute **value** that can be socially described, and that this value is determined by more than individual preference. Coming up with shared moral values means prioritizing according to some standard, and the process of ethical reflection can be described as the application of these standards to do good in the world. Kant says, "Act only on that maxim whereby thou canst at the same time will that it should become a universal law."

A deontological criticism of consequentialism is that an act motivated by the most evil of intentions could by accident produce the most desirable of consequences. If we limited the focus of our attention to an evaluation of the consequences produced by such an action, we would miss an important element of the act and our evaluation would be incomplete.

Both consequentialism and deontology can be criticized because neither offers a final definition of "good consequences" or "right intentions" applicable and readily translatable to the kinds of dilemmas that come to the ethics committee, which is where skill and experience become a critical ingredient of a well-functioning IEC.

Virtue or Character-Based Ethical Thinking:

While consequentialism and deontology look at the action, its consequences, and the intention behind it, the virtue-based approach focuses instead on the agent, and the kind of person the agent is. The focus here is on the person who acts. Aristotle is the main proponent of this school of thought. He talked about acting based on the kind of person one wants to be; if the actor is in the habit of acting a certain way, over time he or she will internalize the virtuous behavior and thereby become a virtuous person.

The starting point here is the identification and selection of a virtuous person who will serve as the standard. When confronted with a difficult dilemma, the critical question is then aimed not at anticipating consequences or uncovering intentions, but rather at what the virtuous person would do.

In the case of the premature, brain damaged newborn, for example, the virtue-based perspective might ask what actions would best express the characteristics that we, as providers, believe are what we want to be — that is are we compassionate, faithful, and so on. The consequentialist may decide to withdraw or withhold treatment, because of the consequences of treatment to the infant, family and society at large; the deontologist may well decide we owe the infant the basic support we provide anyone else. The virtue-based perspective will consider the characteristics of the individuals involved in the dilemma.

As with consequentialism and deontology, some argue that the virtue-based approach is flawed in that there's no standard for deciding what is a "virtuous" person. What if you model yourself on someone who isn't "virtuous," or someone who isn't "virtuous" by another's standards? Of course, Aristotle has much to say about the characteristics of the virtuous person that make him or her universally recognizable. But in contemporary times, and given our cultural diversity, things might not be as clear.

For reasons discussed above, each of these schools of ethical thought can take us only so far when trying to decide what is the best thing to do. But taken together, they provide a starting point for deliberation. For many men and women new to an IEC and ethical deliberation within a clinical context, questions about what is best or right can seem overwhelming; possible answers may all seem relative. A starting point that begins with these three approaches and the understanding that each provides insights and each has weaknesses, can be invaluable in overcoming this initial sense of paralysis.

Beyond a starting point, throughout any ethical deliberation, it's important to know the implications of buying into any one school of thinking, and what follows from it. It's important to know there are many approaches to a problem, and to be able to recognize when only one approach is being brought to bear on a problem. Thus the important question, "Yes, but, have you considered *this*?" can be asked.

Not only are there different schools of ethical reflection, there are also different methodological approaches from which to draw. These include **casuistry,** or the "case-based" approach, and the **principle-based** approach, by far the best known approach to ethical reflection.

Casuistry: The practice of casuistry does not start from general principles and deduce specific answers, but rather begins with the case, and tries to determine where this case fits in with others already seen. In neonatology, for example, where prior directives are nonexistent, this approach is useful in determining whether to withhold or withdraw treatment: we consider the case in relation to previous cases in which decisions have already been made, and see which cases it most closely resembles. This can provide a guide for decision making. Over time and after many cases, IECs develop a "sense," in other words, certain maxims and rules for decision making. Professionals who are more clinically based have a bias toward this casuistic approach, with experience leading their choices. They tend to be consequentialists, or adhere to the virtue-based tradi-

casuistry

tion. They'll develop principles out of their case review experience.

Principle-Based Approach: When considering a specific dilemma, ethical theorists have tended to operate deductively, applying these principles to the dilemma to see if they shed any light. The principles aren't absolute in this approach, nor does any one principle "trump" the others; rather, all these principles provide a repertoire from which to draw specific tools that might be most applicable in specific cases. ☐

Bioethical Principles

Theorists who use the principle-based approach have derived a number of bioethical principles which help us respond to the specific dilemmas faced in clinical settings, despite the diversity of moral traditions from which they may derive. These bioethical principles include **beneficence/nonmaleficence**, **autonomy**, **justice**, and **veracity and fidelity**.

Beneficence and Nonmaleficence:

These companion values derive directly from the consequentialist school and the idea that one should maximize the benefits for the patient, and minimize the harms; these companion values look specifically at outcomes, and perhaps their earliest expression is the Hippocratic Oath and the mandate: "First of all, do no harm."

Nonmaleficence is not the mirror image of beneficence, however. Rather, it's qualitatively different and says that "I have a responsibility to try to protect the patient and will refrain from doing harm, and take great care that the therapies I prescribe and undertake will not inflict undue side effects."

The traditional model of the physician/patient relationship is one in which trust is fundamental. But for that relationship to work, there must also be harmony between the patient's and the physician's notions about what is "harm" and what is "good." Differences between the patient, the healthcare team and the patient's family, as well as differences among the healthcare team about how "harm" and "good" should be weighted and evaluated are the sources of many of the dilemmas an IEC will encounter.

"First of all, do no harm. This is the basic principle derived from the Hippocratic tradition. If we can't benefit someone, then at least we should do that person no harm."

— Tom L. Beauchamp and James Childress, *Principles of Biomedical Ethics*

The fundamental question is whose definition counts, and how should the IEC respond when the case before it arises from such a disagreement? The idea that the healthcare team knows best what constitutes "good" for the patient — paternalism — has limits, as does the beneficence/non-maleficence model, which brings us to *autonomy*.

Autonomy:

The concept of **autonomy** derives from the deontological school of thought which emphasizes duty and acting from the right intentions. One of those right intentions involves treating people with respect, which leads directly to the concept of autonomy, or respecting the capacity and right of rational agents to self-determination.

The term "autonomy" comes from two Greek words: "auto" (self) and "nomos" (law). Together, they mean self-rule, self-determination, self-legislation, or self-definition.

In a clinical setting, autonomy applies to patients who are seen to have the right to self-determination when it comes to deciding what is "harmful" or "beneficial" in treatment.

When the patient's determination differs from that of the caregivers, the question may arise: "Is this person confused? Does he or she have the **capacity** to determine what is 'harmful' and what is 'beneficial' in his or her case?" We'll deal with the concepts of **capacity** and **competency** shortly; for now, suffice it to say that even when capacity and competency may be in question, the starting point for an IEC's consideration is always the patient's autonomy, and some way must always be found to respect that autonomy. This basic principle is supported now by considerable case law throughout the nation.

But how does the concept of autonomy derive from the deontological perspective, and what does this imply for caregivers and for IEC members who will be facing dilemmas raised by clashes between patient autonomy and caregiver paternalism? How, in other words, do we make this concept real in our dealings with others?

Kant said we start by always treating others as individual ends in themselves and never as "mere means." If we treat others as "mere means," then we're using them and controlling them for our purposes, a violation of their right to self-rule and self-determine. From the caregiver's standpoint, then, one doesn't want to treat the patient as a "mere means" to the fulfillment of his or her own goal of doing what he or she considers "good," nor does one want to "use" a patient or case to enhance his or her own reputation. From the resident's viewpoint, one doesn't want to use a patient as a means toward gaining experience and skills. From the manager's viewpoint, one never wants to treat a patient as a means to cost-containment or profitability.

Kant made a qualification here, however. He talked about not using others as *mere* means. Kant recognized that we all "use" others in daily discourse, that we are all means to one another's ends. But in doing so, Kant said, we must not use them as *mere* means, as means only, but recognize that there is something else about that person that's important.

For the National Commission for the Protection of Human Subjects in Biomedical and Behavioral Research in the '70s, these nuances were crucial; human subjects of experiments would indeed be means to an end — the development of new drugs and techniques — but this would be justified only if experimenters also recognized they weren't mere tools.

Another aspect of the concept of autonomy derives from John Stuart Mill. Mill said that we have to respect the right of others not to be interfered with, that we have to respect their right to be left alone and move about in the world as they see fit, as they define their own destinies. He recognized this wasn't an absolute right, of course; the right has boundaries: we have the right not to be interfered with as long as our actions don't pose a direct threat of serious harm to others.

Mill gave an example of this right to noninterference that's useful for clinicians. Suppose you're walking across a bridge and come upon someone standing on the railing about to jump to certain death. Do you have the right to interfere and stop that person? Mill says there is a "limited intervention" that's permissible. You can stop the person and engage him in conversation to help him think about all the implications of his act, and establish that he has the capacity to understand those implications. You may even take advantage of the opportunity to persuade the potential suicide to consider other solutions to his or her problem. After that, however, according to Mill, you have to step back and let the person do what he or she wishes.

There's a certain paternalism that "creeps" into Mill's scheme, however; in stopping the person on the bridge to engage him in conversation, you're assuming he hasn't already thought things through.

Another aspect of "paternalism" appears in emergency rooms; when a patient is brought to an ER in need of immediate help, treatment is given at once on the assumption that once the patient is stabilized, he or she can make

"Over himself, over his own body and mind, the individual is sovereign."

— J.S. Mill, *On Liberty*

in the ER

decisions about continuing care, at which point his or her decisions must be heeded, even if that decision is to withhold or withdraw treatment.

Clearly, the concept of autonomy is not absolute. Like any principle, it has limits, and it does not exist in isolation. The concept of autonomy is closely linked to other concepts in bioethics. For example, Edmund Pellegrino, in his book *The Virtuous Physician*, points out that the physician should respect patient autonomy because it's the beneficent thing to do.

In the clinical setting, autonomy encompasses a give and take between patient and caregiver, and in fact the caregiver's own autonomy or **integrity** can become an issue. Each caregiver, like each patient, is an individual moral agent. He or she has a set of beliefs, values and commitments, and to ask the caregiver to act against them is a violation of his or her **integrity**. Thus the physician has a right to refuse to treat a patient if to do so would violate his or her own beliefs about what is "right" in that case. But a condition of exercising that right is accepting the obligation to transfer that patient's care to another not burdened by such conflicts.

The most fundamental right derived from the right to self-rule and self-determination is the right to determine what happens to our own bodies, and this right is captured in the process of **informed consent** or **informed refusal**; one can't truly determine what should be done with one's body without being fully informed of the implications of any decision and without having a full understanding of those implications.

Informed Consent and Informed Refusal: Informed consent has its roots in a 1914 New York Court of Appeals decision

provider integrity

informed consent and informed refusal

(Schloendorff v. Society of New York Hospital). In that decision, Justice Cardozo wrote that a surgeon who performs surgery on a patient without that patient's *informed* consent commits an assault for which he is liable. Not only does a patient have the right to consent to being treated (consent to "laying on of hands"), but the patient has the right to understand *why* a certain treatment is being proposed, and on the basis of that understanding, give informed consent or refusal.

In essence, the judicial doctrine of informed consent holds that a patient's right of autonomy, to decide what happens to his or her own body, can only be exercised if the information to make a decision is available. It's important to understand that informed consent is not something that happens when the patient signs on the dotted line. Rather, informed consent is a *process* that occurs between the patient and physician within the therapeutic context, or between the physician and patient's surrogates if the patient is incompetent or lacks decision-making capacity.

There are several basic conditions that must be met for consent to be informed and valid: (1) there must be a physician's recommendation with full disclosure of risks, benefits, and alternatives; (2) there must be patient understanding, or the understanding of a surrogate if the patient is incompetent or lacks decision-making capacity; (3) and the resulting consent or refusal must be voluntary and not coerced. Often the cases that will come before the IEC result when one or more of these conditions are not met.

Full Disclosure: In order for the patient to make a fully informed consent, full disclosure must occur about the course of treatment, including all the risks, benefits and alternatives, as well as the implications of refusing treatment. The physician must disclose the diagnosis, and the prognosis. One area of disclosure that commonly leads to problems occurs when the patient is terminally ill and the physician doesn't disclose the prognosis for fear of what effect the knowledge might have on the patient. But again, the patient cannot make an informed consent without knowing the prognosis.

Recommendation: Disclosure alone is not enough, however. Part of the process of informed consent includes the **physician's recommendation**. This is very important. Unfortunately, in an effort not to be "paternalistic" physicians will sometimes avoid making a recommendation, but rather will offer "options". They'll go through a laundry list of risks and benefits, and then say "it's your decision, you decide." But we're talking about informed *consent*, not informed "choice." For the process of informed *consent* to be complete, the patient must be able to consent to — or refuse — a specific recommendation made by the attending physician.

Quite often, it's at this point that the process of informed consent breaks down, and the case finds its way to the IEC. One of the things the IEC will have to determine at the outset is whether the case is there because the physician failed to make a recommendation, resulting in the patient not fully understanding the risks, benefits and alternatives. No dilemma may be involved in such a case, and in fact it may be possible to resolve the issue by suggesting the physician go back and make a clear recommendation.

Patient Understanding: The patient's understanding is an important component of informed consent, and again, understanding isn't complete without the physician's recommendation. Likewise, the caregivers can't be sure that understanding is complete without engaging in the *process* of informed consent, which involves disclosure, checks on understanding, more disclosure and further checks on understanding.

Is Consent or Refusal Voluntary? Another issue that the IEC will have to determine is what factors may be influencing a patient's choice; informed consent presupposes that the consent is **voluntary**, that no coercion was involved. Is the family exerting undue influence on the patient, for instance? Do they make it impossible for the physician to talk openly and privately with the patient about the risks and benefits of a proposed intervention?

Capacity and Competence: Two critically important concepts — capacity and competence — are embedded in this sketch of the conditions that make an informed consent process successful. That is, we have presumed that the patient engaged in the informed consent process has the capacity and the competency to understand information as it is disclosed, and voluntarily consents to or refuses the proposed treatment. But what if the patient lacks the capacity necessary to fully participate in the process? To address this kind of case, IEC members must understand the difference between the related but distinct concepts of **capacity** and **competency**.

Competence is a legal status. In our society, one is assumed to be competent if over 18, unless a judge specifically declares otherwise. **Capacity** is judged clinically, and has to do with whether or not the patient is capable of understanding the options presented. Thus a 15-year-old patient and a 90-year-old patient can present quite distinct

Is consent or refusal voluntary?

capacity and competence

Competence is a legal judgment... capacity is a clinical judgment.

problems in terms of competency and capacity. The young patient is not legally competent, but it's probably safe for caregivers to assume he or she is fully capable of understanding a treatment course, and making informed decisions about it, though not legally competent to give consent.

The 90-year-old, perhaps with questionable capacity, may still be legally competent, but not reliably capable of understanding and making informed decisions about his or her care. IEC members must be sensitive to the distinctions between capacity and competency, that in some cases the patient might be quite capable of understanding and participating in decisions about treatment regardless what his or her legal status may be, and that those decisions carry considerable moral weight.

Capacity is not an either/or proposition, unfortunately; there are nuances to capacity, different *layers* of capacity that will complicate any deliberation. The differences can be likened to concentric circles, or to the skins of an onion. The outermost layer is the capacity to make decisions about work and business life; next, family life; then daily routine; and the inner-most, most fundamental capacity concerns the making of decisions about one's own body, to say "touch me" or "don't."

In the clinical setting, the concept of informed consent frequently is concerned with this most fundamental of capacities. It may well be that the patient is not capable any longer of making decisions about business, family life or daily routine due to illness, medications or other factors. Caregivers and IEC members must consider whether that same patient is nonetheless still capable of making decisions about his or her own body, and care-givers must do so without making assumptions based on possible other incapacities. Conditions such as depression and changing one's mind, for example, could at first glance seem to be symptoms of incapacity, but this may not necessarily be so. Caregivers must also make a distinction between **decisional capacity** and **executional capacity** (the capacity to carry out a decision). A paraplegic may not be able to carry out decisions, but he or she may nonetheless be fully capable of making those decisions.

There is national consensus on the issue of autonomy as reflected in court cases nationwide; case law fully supports the *competent* patient's right to make decisions about his or her own care, including refusing treatment or demanding that treatment be discontinued, even when the caregivers believe the treatment is in the patient's best interest.

Some have argued that there are exceptions to the principle of autonomy, for example when there is a need to protect innocent third parties — when a single mother of young children refuses, for religious reasons, a blood transfusion vital to her survival. This is an area of intense debate right now, and the question of whether individuals give up some religious freedoms simply because they're parents is coming under increasing scrutiny in both the literature and in recent court decisions (please refer to Legal Issues).

Problems occur, and case law state by state differs, when the patient is no longer competent or never was. Then questions about surrogacy and what is a "legitimate surrogate" are raised. States may also differ on how much disclosure is necessary in such cases, as well as what are the standards any "reasonable" person would expect to constitute full disclosure. Check with hospital counsel regarding court decisions that may be relevant in your area.

Formerly Competent Patients: What happens when a formerly healthy man or woman lapses into coma, or becomes incapable of understanding or making decisions about care, perhaps due to a disease such as Alzheimer's?

We recognize the capacity and right of people to go through the informed consent and informed refusal process, and *that right continues and endures through a loss of capacity.* It would be meaningless to say that a patient with capacity has this right, but loses it once he or she lapses into incapacity.

The task, then, is to ascertain what the formerly capable person wanted. If the patient left some written directive in the form of a "living will" or durable power of attorney for healthcare, for example, outlining acceptable levels of care or no "extraordinary" measures, the matter is reasonably clear, and caregivers must abide by that directive (we'll get to the matter of what is "extraordinary" on page 91).

In the absence of such a written directive, we look for a **substituted judgment** from a surrogate, someone who can stand in place of the patient and give voice to what the patient would want to say, if the patient had the capacity. If the patient left a Durable Power of Attorney designating someone to speak for him or her, then it's clear. If the patient hasn't, then the IEC must dig deeper in search of someone who can exercise a best-interests judgment, usually a family member or close friend.

It's important that everyone involved in such a case be quite clear about the difference between judgments concerning the patient's **best interests** and **substituted judgments**.

Consider the case of a Parkinson's patient who has suffered severe head trauma from a fall. He has an intracranial bleed and the surgeons want to operate to relieve the pressure, otherwise he'll die. However, the patient has two daughters who differ widely concerning what level of care should be provided. One wants surgery for her father, the other asks that it not be done. When questioned, the daughter who wants treatment says "I think it would be best for him to have the surgery." The other daughter says, "I don't think this is what Dad would have wanted. I think Dad was tired of living with his disability, and would want to die."

The first daughter is offering a **best interests argument** in favor of surgery; the other is attempting to speak for her father and tell the committee what he would want, a **substituted judgment.** The IEC will have to take other factors into consideration, of course (please see "Methodology" for a detailed description of this process), including possible conflicts of interest, but in general, if there is evidence of the patient's wishes, the second daughter's argument for what her *father* would want carries more weight. Whenever an IEC hears nurses, physicians or a patient's family talking about what *they* think is best in such a case, the IEC needs to shift the focus conceptually and ask what the *patient* would want, regardless what might be clinically "best"; did he or she ever say anything to anyone about the sort of care desired? Did he or she ever write anything?

Never Competent, Not Yet Competent, or Incompetent Patients With No Identifiable Surrogates: This class of patients poses particularly difficult problems. The never competent patient, perhaps a severely retarded adult, or the not yet competent patient, a baby, will not have communicated preferences, or developed an identifiable value system, so it's pointless for caregivers or family to ask what the patient would want. There's no way for them to know.

The only choice we have in such cases is to consider what is in the patient's **best interests**. Commonly, such cases center on a newborn; in these cases, we look to the parents for guidance as to the baby's best interest, on the assumption that the parents have the closest bond and their decisions are the most trustworthy.

Another common situation involves a homeless person brought into the ER; the patient has no family, no friends, no support network to speak for him or to help in a best interest judgment. In these cases the attending physician will often bring the matter to the IEC in order not to "play God," but to involve others in the decision about what is in the patient's best interest.

Justice:

The principle of justice is broad, overarching and, like concepts such as "love," so vague that it's difficult to discuss meaningfully. Still, we appeal to the principle all the time when considering what it would mean to treat individuals fairly, either in the context of therapeutic relationships, or in the context of institutional or public policy. A general rule derived from Aristotle is that treating individuals fairly means treating equals equally and unequals unequally. In other words, all other things being equal in terms of diagnosis and prognosis, all metastatic breast cancer patients should receive the same treatment options, regardless of such factors as personal qualities and financial status.

The idea is that making a commitment to treating equals equally and unequals unequally guards against arbitrary decision-making and promotes consistent and impartial decisions instead.

This is not to say that a commitment to fairness always leads to clear-cut answers. It may be difficult to determine what it would mean to treat equals equally since there isn't always agreement about the sense in which individuals need to be equal in order to be treated equally. Still, the principle of justice helps frame the parameters within which the right questions can be asked.

The scope of the principle's application doesn't end with a commitment to treating equals equally. Justice also addresses more global questions such as the proper distribution and allocation of scarce resources. And, as IEC members will soon discover, rare is the case that comes to the committee that doesn't raise a question of justice at this level, be it the allocation of time, money, staff, beds or equipment.

Like any other question of values, there are a variety of approaches to the dilemmas posed by scarce resources, and the IEC members should familiarize themselves with the different positions represented in the current debate. We suggest that most questions of justice as they arise in cases of scarce resources are better addressed at the policy level than at the bedside. In this regard, the IEC will have to decide what issues it *will* be willing to entertain, and in what contexts.

Veracity and Fidelity:

These principles cover the issues of truth-telling, promise-keeping and confidentiality. **Veracity** and **fidelity** are implied in the requirements of justice in any relationship between two people. Ethical theorists and philosophers in general talk about the necessity for truth-telling and commitment; here, we're focusing on the requirements of a specific kind of relationship, that between a professional and a client, or still more specifically, between a physician or other health professional and the patient.

There has been an ancient tradition in the ethics of medicine from the time of Hippocrates that the best way to define a relationship between a physician and patient is in terms of **professional paternalism** (a preferable, non-sexist term would be **"parentalism"**), that the professional has a fiduciary responsibility, once entering into the relationship, to care for and be responsible *for* (not *to*) the patient, as a parent would be for a child. In this formulation, both expert knowledge and wisdom are required, that is, the capacity to make good decisions on the patient's behalf.

Veracity: In order for the patient and physician to enter into such a relationship, there must be a climate of trust; the patient must trust that the physician is technically competent and working in his or her best interests. For trust to exist, the physician must tell the truth — **veracity** — and the patient must have the *expectation* that the physician will always tell the truth.

A classic example of an inappropriate or unjustified paternalism is the physician who decides not to tell a patient he's terminally ill. There has been intense debate, particularly between the world wars, over this issue: should the physician *always* tell the truth to a patient, or withhold the truth to protect the patient from the consequences of knowledge, just as a parent might withhold the truth from a child? The debate has cooled considerably; at this point in history, there is general consensus that patients should always be told the truth.

Fidelity says that irrespective of payment, the expectation of payment, or the personal qualities of the patient, the physican will maintain that initial commitment to provide care for the patient. Like veracity, fidelity is inherent in the concept of paternalism: just as a parent presumably does not abandon the child when the child becomes inconvenient, obnoxious or ill, likewise the physician is expected to maintain a relationship with the patient once the relationship has begun.

Indeed, statutory law in the U.S. requires that once a physician enters into a relationship with a patient, he or she can only remove himself or herself from the case if a transfer can be made to a physician of comparable skill who is willing to take over the patient's care. This is a concrete example of fidelity, and this standard enables patients to trust that they won't be abandoned if they happen to challenge their physician in some way.

Veracity and fidelity are what we call "operational" principles. The companion principles of beneficence/nonmaleficence are more related to the "content" of acts and decisions. The principle of autonomy stands against paternalism, and redefines the entire physician/patient relationship as a contractual one between equals. □

SPECIAL CONSIDERATIONS

Withholding and Withdrawing Treatment: While withdrawing a treatment from a patient might "feel" different than simply withholding it, by all standards the two are considered equal; there is no ethical or legal difference between withholding and withdrawing treatment. In a clinical setting, we never believe that an intervention, once started, can't be stopped. Rather, we'll try a treatment, see if it works, and if it doesn't, withdraw it and try something else, or stop treatment entirely. In the ER in particular, treatments are begun all the time in order to stabilize the patient, with the understanding that you're "buying time" to decide what's best. The family considering the withdrawal of life support may have a hard time accepting the idea that withholding and withdrawal are morally equal, however, and the IEC will want to help them understand this point when the issue is part of a dilemma under consideration.

The issue of withholding or withdrawing treatment when a "best interest" or substituted judgment is being made is more complex than when a competent patient is making the decision. In the case of a patient in a persistent vegetative state, for example, decisions about withholding or withdrawing treatment will contain elements of best interest judgments, as well as a search for insights into the patient's previously expressed wishes. Hopefully, when providers have to make best interest judgments, they do so in the context of whatever values the patient held, rather than sitting on the "outside" and making judgments about quality of life.

Proportionality/Usefulness vs. Ordinary/Extraordinary: When considering whether to withhold or withdraw care, the question is often asked if the care being considered is "ordinary" or "extraordinary" care. Many patient directives specify no "extraordinary" care, for example, while caregivers often feel obligated to provide "ordinary" care.

But there has been a conceptual shift in healthcare away from considerations about **ordinary/extraordinary** toward considerations about **proportionality** and **usefulness.** The previously established standards for determining what was "ordinary" care looked at whether or not the care was technologically simple, "standard operating procedure," commonly done, and "natural." If the intervention was *not* any of these things, then it was considered extraordinary and therefore caregivers were not obligated to provide it.

The problem with these standards first of all is that they didn't consider the specific intervention in the context of a particular patient's situation; these standards didn't ask if the intervention was ordinary or extraordinary for *this* particular patient.

Another problem was that what was once technologically complex, rare and "unnatural" might now be quite common and routine; the ventilator, for example, was extraordinary care not too long ago; today it's ordinary.

With the growing recognition of the limits of the ordinary/extraordinary standards, we're moving toward a more nuanced approach. First, we ask whether the intervention would be **disproportionately burdensome** to the patient, causing more harm or pain than benefit in curing or restoring function. The advantage here is that caregivers must weigh the benefits and burdens of an intervention for a *particular patient*.

The next consideration is how **useful** is the intervention? That is, how likely is it to produce the desired results? This particular issue is a can of worms right now, however; the issue of **futility** is the subject of considerable and heated debate in the healthcare community, and as yet no definition of futility has been proposed that everyone can live with. The stumbling block here is that we have to ask "futile in terms of *what*?" Is an intervention futile in terms of a specific goal? What is that goal? To prolong life? To restore quality of life? Or is the goal something clear and clinical, the restoration of electrolyte balance, for instance? Who decides the goal? The issue of futility spans a spectrum running from simple physiologic futility to questions of value: is it *worth* it?

In any case, the assessments of benefits, burdens and usefulness are made by the healthcare team, and these assessments are then brought into the informed consent process with the competent patient, or the surrogate who's making a substituted judgment for the incompetent patient, or with whomever is going to make a best interest judgment for the never or not yet competent patient.

Among the healthcare team, there are likely to be different views about what is a benefit or burden for a particular patient, or what is going to be "useful" or "futile" in that case. There are also likely to be differences among family members, and between the family and providers, and it's these disagreements that give rise to the IEC case consultation, and with which you'll have to deal. ☐

The issue of futility spans a spectrum running from simple physiologic futility to questions of value: is it worth *it?*

Suggested Readings

• Tom L. Beauchamp, **Philosophical Ethics**. McGraw Hill, 1982.

• Tom L. Beauchamp, **Principles of Biomedical Ethics** (3rd ed.). Oxford University Press, 1989.

• Tom L. Beauchamp and LeRoy Walters, eds., **Contemporary Issues in Bioethics**. Wadsworth Publishing Company, 1989.

• Baruch Brody, **Life and Death Decision Making**. Oxford University Press, 1988.

• Allen E. Buchanan and Dan W. Brock, **Deciding for Others: the Ethics of Surrogate Decision Making**. Cambridge University Press, 1989.

• Edmund D. Pellegrino and David C. Thomasma, **For the Patient's Good: the Restoration of Beneficence in Health Care**. Oxford University Press, 1988.

• Paul S. Appelbaum, W. Charles and Alan Meisel, **Informed Consent: Legal Theory and Clinical Practice**. Oxford University Press, 1987.

• James F. Childress, **Who Should Decide? Paternalism in Health Care**. Oxford University Press, 1982.

• Jay Katz, **The Silent World of Doctor and Patient**. Macmillan Press, 1984.

• **Making Health Care Decisions**. President's Commission for the Study of Ethical Problems in Medicine and Biomedical and Behavioral Research, U.S. Government Printing Office, 1982-83.

LEGAL ISSUES

Introduction

The committee does not assume that law provides an answer to every question, nor that law is the most relevant source of answers.

Because of our society's diversity, we sometimes assume that the law is the only authority which commonly will be acknowledged when claims or values are in conflict. In part this is so because the law is backed by the power of the state. This can lead to fear of the law by some people, including members of ethics committees. In addition, we have grown familiar over the last thirty years or more with having difficult issues — i.e. civil rights and the environment — resolved in the legislatures and the courts. This has led some to assume that the legal system is the appropriate forum to resolve *all* conflicts in values.

An ethics committee offers a different method to resolve conflicting values in a healthcare setting. For the healthy ethics committee, the law is only one of many factors to consider. The committee does not assume that law provides an answer to every question, nor that law is the most relevant source of answers. Learning about the law is a necessary step in liberating the committee process from undue legal influence because:

First: Familiarity with the legal system and relevant law can reduce the possibility that members' fears and concerns about the law will "chill" the committee's work. An understanding of the law and its boundaries will free the members to address the ethics of clinical cases in confidence. The committee needs enough familiarity with the legal system to understand what guidance the law can — and can't — provide in the committee's work. More generally, the committee will want to be familiar with the applicable law with regard to **informed consent, withdrawal/withholding of treatment,** and other subjects which arise frequently in the committee's work. Such knowledge will help to keep legal concerns separate from ethical concerns.

Second: Learning about the law will help calm members' fears of personal exposure to lawsuits arising out of their ethics committee work. To the best of our knowledge, no one has ever been successfully sued for his or her work on an ethics committee. This is not surprising when we remember that an ethics committee does not make decisions; it makes recommendations which others can then choose to follow or not.

In a society in which anyone with the filing fee can bring a lawsuit against anyone else, no one can offer absolute assurance that members of an ethics committee never will be named in a lawsuit. For this reason it is appropriate that the committee's institutional sponsor arrange for the indemnification of the members. However, members can be assured that good ethics makes good law. Exposure to personal legal liability as a result of good faith participation in an ethics committee is very remote.

Third: Becoming familiar with case law can be useful as an analytic tool. The previous chapter on ethical theory discussed some of the approaches to ethical analysis. One of these approaches, which has been the focus of revived interest in recent years, is **casuistry**. In this approach to ethics, ethical analysis begins not with general principles from which answers are deduced, but rather with specific cases for which there is consensus concerning the appropriate outcome. An ethics consultation involving the comparison of the facts presented with those of other cases in order to determine the best recommendation under the circumstances is casuistic; an essential element in the casuistic approach is to identify cases within a taxonomy which are most analogous to the case under consideration. Therefore, studying legal precedent for its reasoning as well as for its outcome can facilitate the use of the casuistic method in the committee's work. ☐

Exposure to personal legal liability as a result of good faith participation in an ethics committee is very remote.

ETHICS COMMITTEES AND THE LAW

S everal questions frequently asked by those becoming familiar with the work of ethics committees include:

- How does law relate to ethics?
- If something is illegal, is it unethical by definition?
- If ethics is a process rather than a set of answers or values, is it necessary for an ethics committee to be familiar with legal precedent?
- Can the committee simply do its ethical analysis and let others (risk managers and lawyers, for example) worry about the legal implications?

In this section, we'll seek to answer these and other law-related questions which may arise in the work of an ethics committee.

Law, morals and ethics — there is a difference

In the previous chapter on ethical theory, morality was distinguished from ethics. Morality was described as a belief about what is best to do, based upon a consensus of values and an authority to which one can turn in particular cases. The law is an expression of morality, with respect to some subjects. The legal prohibition against murder no doubt reflects society's consensus that murder is wrong. In fact, the strength of the moral consensus that murder is wrong underlies the official rule against murder and places the power of the state behind its enforcement.

However, not all illegal acts are immoral. The legal

prohibition in the United States against driving on the left side of the street is simply a convention designed to facilitate orderly transportation. It does not represent a societal consensus that driving on the left is intrinsically immoral. In this respect, law is driven by a consequentialist argument — everyone must drive on the same side of the road so as to minimize collisions.

Some commentators have observed that many of the legal restrictions on the withdrawal of treatment have been based upon fear of the consequences, fear that unscrupulous family members occasionally might abuse a patient in a less restricted system. These legal restrictions reflect society's moral conviction that the *class* of powerless people needs to be protected. However, in a *particular* case, a family's good faith may be clearly apparent; in a particular case, it may be clear that a particular patient *is* protected. Under such circumstances, an ethics committee can address the way in which a *particular* person is treated, and the legal requirements may in such circumstances be morally neutral, even though legally enforceable. Does this mean legal restrictions are irrelevant in such cases? Not at all. It does mean that the IEC shouldn't allow itself to be restricted by legal concerns when considering all the options in a particular case when it's clear the patient *is* protected.

Even when a law reflects a genuine societal consensus when it is enacted, such a consensus can erode over time. Since laws can be changed or repealed only through deliberate action, a law may continue to compel or forbid a given activity though there is no longer a moral consensus supporting the law.

Ours is a heterogeneous culture, and society has found it difficult to achieve true consensus on right and wrong with regard to some subjects with which the ethics committee will be occupied. Withholding and withdrawing life-sustaining treatments, balancing the needs of patient confidentiality and risk to others, defining the limits of patient autonomy and the healthcare professional's rights and responsibilities are only a few of the issues with which society and the law have struggled.

Society has reached consensus on several of the issues which ethics committees frequently encounter, and this consensus is being reflected in the law. Respect for the individual's autonomy regarding medical treatment is now generally accepted, morally and legally, for example. Rapidly evolving technologies will ensure, however, that ethics committees will be faced with questions which law either has not answered or which law has answered only partially or imperfectly.

For now, the most that can be said is that the law *sometimes* reflects our society's morality with respect to a particular issue which is implicated in an ethics committee case consultation. However, the law is never a substitute for the committee's process of ethical reflection. Ethics is designed to balance conflicting values. The clinical cases on which ethics committees are consulted typically involve values which are by their nature intensely personal and private. Even when the law actually does express a dominant morality, its application to a *particular* clinical case may not be ethically appropriate. The individual patient, family or healthcare provider may hold values which differ from the dominant morality, and the process of ethical reflection is necessary to resolve such a conflict.

Ethics committees naturally will want to know whether or not a proposed course of action is legal. Although an ethics committee is not engaged in risk management, the legality of a recommendation is part of the terrain to be considered. The process described in Methodology locates where, in the case consultation process, the legal issues specific to a given case are discussed. However, it is crucial that the committee not confuse its ethical deliberation with what is or is not legal.

An Overview of the Legal System

The legal system in the United States can be confusing to those who have never had occasion to become involved in it. Although the system is complex in its totality, members of an ethics committee need concern themselves with only certain aspects of the system.

Most people are aware that ours is a dual legal system comprised of state and national governments. The national government and each state have their own constitutions, legislatures, court systems and regulatory agencies. This federal form of government reflects the desire of those who framed the U.S. Constitution to balance the claims for a strong central government against the competing interests in autonomy for the individual states. As a result of this balance, the national (or Federal) government is limited to those powers allocated to it by the U.S. Constitution. The states' powers extend to all matters not reserved by the Constitution to Federal jurisdiction. Laws can originate within the Federal jurisdiction or a state's jurisdiction in a variety of ways.

The Constitution — One source of law is constitutional, either the U.S. Constitution or a state's constitution. Constitutions guarantee individuals certain rights or freedoms,

the constitution

such as freedom of speech, of religion, and of privacy. A state's constitution may guarantee citizens of that state greater rights than the U.S. Constitution, but a state may not restrict its citizens from enjoying those rights guaranteed by the U.S. Constitution.

The constitutional issue in the case of **Nancy Cruzan** (see below) was whether the State of Missouri, in refusing to permit the withdrawal of nutrition and hydration, had violated the rights of privacy and liberty guaranteed to Nancy Cruzan under the U.S. Constitution. The case was ultimately decided by the U.S. Supreme Court because that court has the final authority to interpret the U.S. Constitution. A state's supreme court has the final say in interpreting that particular state's constitution.

The Legislatures — A second source of law is legislative. Congress' enactment of the Patient Self-Determination Act is an example of legislation which creates a duty to act (in this case the duty of providers to provide information to their patients or the patients' family members, among other things, as a condition to receiving Federal funds). Other legislation does not mandate action but merely is permissive. A number of state legislatures, for example, have passed statutes concerning surrogate decision-making (durable powers of attorney for healthcare, or "health proxies"). Such statutes have clarified, and in some cases created, the ability of individuals to ensure that their wishes regarding medical treatment are respected even if they become incompetent. Such legislation does not require that people appoint surrogates, however.

With the exception of the Patient Self-Determination Act, Congress has left the regulation of surrogate decision making to the state legislatures. Such related matters as

Nancy Cruzan

the legislatures

guardianships and conservatorships have traditionally been matters for state law. The law of surrogate decision-making will probably remain defined by state law, limited only by those individual rights guaranteed by the U.S. Constitution. In other areas of bioethics, however, there may be relevant Federal legislation as well as state statutes.

Regulations — Another source of law related to the legislative are administrative regulations, issued pursuant to authority granted to government agencies by the Congress or state legislatures. Examples of such regulations are the FDA regulations on the protection of those who are research subjects in clinical trials of experimental drugs and devices (which have been embraced generally), and the so-called "Baby Doe" regulations (which have elicited considerable controversy). Federal regulations frequently condition eligibility for Medicare and Medicaid funding on compliance with such regulations. States occasionally have declined to comply with such regulations as originally issued, relying on public pressure to ensure that the regulations were modified or rescinded.

The Courts — A fourth source of law are the courts. Courts express law through the decisions they hand down on particular cases and the opinions which usually (although not always) accompany those decisions. Although a court decision literally decides only the particular dispute which has been presented by the facts of the case, court decisions have been instrumental in shaping the conduct of all of society by the principles announced in the opinions underlying those decisions.

Court decisions take several forms. A court may issue orders (often called injunctions) or award money damages or dismiss a plaintiff's claim. In criminal cases a court may convict a defendant of a crime (resulting in incarceration or fines) or acquit the defendant. Appeals courts' decisions take the form of affirming (upholding), reversing or modifying a lower court's decision. The famous cases of <u>Quinlan</u> and <u>Cruzan</u> each involved whether or not the court should issue an order authorizing the withdrawal of certain medical interventions. <u>Schloendorff</u> v. <u>Society of New York Hospital</u>, addressing the issue of informed consent, arose out of a patient's attempt to recover money damages for her hospital treatment. An important California case <u>Barber v. Superior Court</u>, is one of the few bioethics cases involving criminal law. The <u>Barber</u> decision involved whether or not a criminal prosecution of two physicians would be allowed to proceed.

A decision may be based largely upon an interpretation of a constitutional provision or of a particular statute or regulation. In other cases the issues raised may be governed by what is called the "common law". Historically, common law was only one of two systems of principles used by courts ("equity" being the other). Today the distinction between the two systems has lost its practical significance to nonlawyers, and the common law generally refers to the collection of prior judicial opinions which has gained respect and authority through the test of time. The common law finds its roots in legal decisions in medieval England and continues its evolution today.

For example, the legal concept of informed consent developed from the common law. Faced with a patient's complaint against a hospital at being treated medically without permission, the judge in <u>Schloendorff</u> considered prior legal decisions for an analogy. He concluded that the common law concept of trespass was analogous to being treated without consent. That analogy subsequently gained general acceptance in other courts and jurisdictions, and the doctrine of informed consent is now a firmly established principle of American common law. It did not happen overnight, however. To understand why, law as an evolutionary process must be understood.

Holdings and Dicta — An opinion is a judge's way of explaining the reasoning which led to the decision in a particular case. Those principles which are *necessary* to reach the decision are called the **"holding"** of the case. Were these principles different, in other words, a different decision logically would be necessary. Frequently an opinion will announce or endorse other principles as well, which are not *necessary* to reach the decision, but which the judge feels are relevant to the issues raised in the case. These principles are called **"dicta."**

For example, in <u>Schloendorff</u>, the court upheld a verdict in favor of the hospital, holding that a charitable hospital was not responsible for the acts of physicians practicing there. That was the court's "holding", because in 1914 that was the prevailing law. Since the physicians had not been sued, the court did not need to discuss whether they should have asked the patient's permission before operating on her. However, the "dicta," that every adult and competent person has a right to determine what will be done with his or her own body, was ground-breaking and is what makes the case relevant today.

The Authority of Courts — Court cases may be authoritative in two different senses. The United States, the District of Columbia and the fifty states each has an ultimate court to which appeals may be taken. These courts are usually,

holdings

dicta

although not always, called supreme courts. In their respective jurisdictions the decisions of these courts are binding upon lower courts. For example, the California supreme court is the ultimate arbiter with respect to California common law as well as interpreting the California constitution and California statutes and regulations. However, if a California statute is challenged as a violation of the U.S. Constitution, the U.S. Supreme Court is the ultimate authority.

The second sense in which a court's decision may be authoritative is in its persuasive power, and it is in this sense that "dicta" are authoritative. The clarity of reasoning displayed by an opinion may influence other courts in the same jurisdiction and in other jurisdictions, even though they are not bound by the first court's ruling. As court after court reaches the same result in similar cases, a common jurisprudence coalesces. This has occurred in several areas of bioethics, including informed consent, the patient's right to refuse treatment, establishment of the equivalence of withdrawing and withholding treatment, and the consideration of nutrition and hydration as equivalent to other medical interventions.

What is "legal"?

What is "legal" and what is not sometimes is not easily determined. It is worth observing that the differing sources of the law have implications for the very term "legal". Occasionally someone on an ethics committee may ask, "Is option X *legal*?" The preceding discussion of the ways in which the law arises should illustrate how complex such a simple question can be.

Assume, for example, that a case confronting the committee involves the withdrawal of artificial nutrition and hydration from a patient in a persistent vegetative state (PVS). All members of the patient's family agree that the patient's prior expressions and values indicate that she would not want to continue life support under the circumstances. The patient's son has been appointed her guardian, under a state statute that gives him the legal power to make treatment decisions on his mother's behalf, and he has asked the attending physician to discontinue the feeding.

Assume further that the state legislature had passed a "living will" statute. The statute was aimed at ensuring that a competent individual's wishes concerning treatment would be honored after he or she became incompetent, by permitting such an individual to make a written declaration or "living will." In such a document, the individual can specify what treatments should not be administered, depending on particular circumstances. However, one section of the statute excludes food and nourishment as procedures that can be withdrawn under the statutory "living will."

Although the patient never signed such a "living will," does the state statute's prohibition on withdrawal of nutrition and hydration by "living will" imply that a surrogate decison maker (the son in this case) should not be able to order the withdrawal of nutrition and hydration? Would it be illegal to honor the wishes of the patient, as conveyed by the family?

This case actually arose in Hawaii, in the 1990 case of In re Guardianship of Crabtree. The son, who was a lawyer, sought a court's permission to terminate his mother's treatment. The court ruled that the statute was ambiguous, and that in any event the patient had a constitutional right to

*In re Guardianship
of Crabtree*

have the nutrition and hydration removed, notwithstanding the statute. Did the court's ruling answer the question of legality? Since only decisions of the state's appeals courts are binding, another judge in the same state could reach a different conclusion so long as the legislature leaves the statute intact and the supreme court has not settled the question. Some future court might find the statute unambiguous but inapplicable, or unambiguous but unconstitutional, or unambiguous and enforceable. On the other hand, another judge presented with a similar case might well find the first court's decision very persuasive.

The lack of absolute certainty about what is "legal" is one reason ethics committees will want to focus primarily upon ethics and not on law. For despite some members' expectations, the question "What is the law?" all too often will not clarify the issue if posed early in the committee's deliberations. It merely will generate a time consuming and fruitless discussion of various possible arguments. Once the committee has completed its ethical deliberations, it will have sufficiently narrowed the issues so that reference to law will then be more productive. □

A Primer On Relevant Law

Much of the law with which ethics committees need be concerned is state law, and a comprehensive survey of all the law of all fifty states, with respect to even one bioethics issue, would exceed the scope of this work. This section is intended as a beginning resource, with the aim of orienting the reader to general trends in several areas of the law which are important to an ethics committee's work. Each committee will want to become familiar with the relevant statutory and case law in the state in which the committee operates, realizing that on some issues there may not yet be any law.

That said, some of the issues with which the committee will deal have been addressed in a number of jurisdictions. There has arisen a striking consensus among courts with respect to some of these subjects. The following outlines this consensus with regard to several subjects arising around treatment issues.

The Patient's Right To Decide and Surrogate Decision Making

Schloendorff v. Society of New York Hospital — The Schloendorff case, referred to earlier, is only one of the early cases which established the legal obligation of a physician to obtain a patient's consent before performing an operation or other procedure. The earlier section on ethical theory discusses what is involved in obtaining in-formed consent. The patient's right to consent is commonly acknowledged to imply the patient's right to refuse treatment as well. However, this right to control what happens to one's own body never has been absolute.

First, courts have generally limited this right to adults who are competent to make decisions about their treatment. In its discussion of autonomy, the earlier chapter on ethical theory discusses the subject of decision-making capacity. When a court examines an individual's capacity, it is called competence, but the factors considered in determining a person's capacity or competence are the same.

Even competent adults have not always enjoyed the absolute right to refuse treatment. Most of the early cases considering refusal of treatment arose in the context of refusals of treatment based upon religious grounds, often by Jehovah's Witnesses or Christian Scientists. Courts generally came to agree that there were four possible "state interests" in ordering treatment over an individual's objections: 1) a state interest in the preservation of life, 2) a state interest in preventing suicide, 3) a state interest in protecting innocent third parties (usually children), and 4) a state interest in protecting the integrity of the medical profession. Courts weighed these interests against the individual's interest in individual autonomy and bodily integrity.

Among the factors which courts often have used to balance the state's interests against the individual's are the extent to which the treatment would violate firmly held patient values, the degree of the treatment's invasiveness, the prognosis with and without treatment, the existence of persons dependant upon the patient, and the intensity of the health professionals' assertions of their interest in healing. The evaluation of these and other factors by various courts has not been uniform or consistent. Patients' religious and personal beliefs which are not shared by judges and physicians frequently have been given little weight in the balancing process, especially when the treatment at issue was standard medical practice which promised a complete cure.

In re Quinlan — In 1976 the scope of a patient's right to refuse treatment which could not cure was considered in the case of In re Quinlan. Karen Quinlan had suffered brain damage in 1975 which left her in PVS and on a ventilator. Her father sought court permission to take Karen off the ventilator because there was no hope of her eventual recovery. The court refused Mr. Quinlan's request, saying that the nature and extent of care were to be governed by the standards of medical practice, and Karen's physician declined to take her off the respirator. Mr. Quinlan appealed to the New Jersey Supreme Court.

The Supreme Court reversed the lower court and granted Mr. Quinlan permission to have Karen removed from the ventilator. In doing so the court held that Karen had the right to refuse treatment, exercisable through her father, based upon a constitutional right to privacy. The state's interest in preserving life diminished where, as here, the invasiveness of the treatment was great and the prognosis extremely poor.

The court went on to find that the standards of medical practice then existing in New Jersey, which barred the withdrawal of the ventilator, should be reevaluated under the circumstances. The advances of medical technology, the court said, made it necessary to focus on the prognosis of the patient rather than the nature of the intervention itself. The court surmised that one reason the medical profession was reluctant to forgo aggressive treatment of dying patients was the corrosive influence of malpractice litigation and the threat of criminal prosecution. The court endorsed the use of ethics committees as a way of ensuring that all relevant issues were aired in such cases, which would give physicians greater confidence. The court also held that removing Karen from the ventilator would not be homicide, thereby allaying fears of criminal liability.

Lane v. Candura — Since the <u>Quinlan</u> decision, courts in many states have recognized the individual's right to determine his or her medical treatment, including the refusal of treatment. In 1978 a Massachusetts appeals court was faced in <u>Lane v. Candura</u> with a 77 year-old woman with a gangrenous right foot and leg who refused amputation. The court emphasized Mrs. Candura's ability to understand that the consequences of her refusal would be death and held that a competent adult had the right to make her own decision to accept or reject treatment, whether others viewed the decision as wise or not. In reaching its decision, the court relied upon a case decided one year earlier by Massachusetts' highest court, <u>Superintendent of Belchertown State School v. Saikewicz</u>. The court there relied on both the constitutional right to privacy and the common law right to informed consent to permit chemotherapy to be withheld from a profoundly retarded man with leukemia. The court justified its decision on the grounds it was expressing what the patient's wishes would have been had he been competent.

Bartling v. Superior Court — <u>Bartling v. Superior Court</u> presented a California appeals court in 1984 with a case in which a patient refused life sustaining treatment. Mr. Bartling was a 70 year-old who was placed on a respirator following the collapse of a lung during a biopsy on a tumor. Suffering from emphysema, Mr. Bartling could not be weaned from the respirator and demanded that it be disconnected, even though he acknowledged he would die as a result. He preferred death to life through mechanical means. However, the hospital and his treating physicians refused to disconnect the ventilator, saying such an act would violate their medical integrity. They also expressed fear of civil or criminal liability, since the patient was not terminally ill. Although the hospital was willing to transfer Mr. Bartling to another facility, none could be found.

The appeals court held that the right to refuse treatment was not limited to terminally ill patients or to those in a coma. All competent adults have that right, the court said, based upon the constitutional right of privacy. The court went on to observe that "if the right of the patient to self determination as to his own medical care is to have any meaning at all, it must be paramount to the interests of the patient's hospital and doctors." The court discounted any fears that carrying out a patient's instructions could lead to civil or criminal liability, saying that no state interests outweighed Mr. Bartling's interest in his own treatment.

Bouvia v. Superior Court — Two years later another California court of appeals, in <u>Bouvia v. Superior Court</u>, sustained a 28-year-old woman suffering from severe cerebral palsy in her demand that a nasogastric feeding tube be removed. Her physicians feared that without the tube Ms. Bouvia would not be able to take enough nutrition to live; in fact, it was argued, her refusal to consent to tube feeding was an attempt at suicide, which the state had an interest in preventing. The court responded by distinguishing between a patient who wishes to die and a patient who is willing to accept death when continued life can be purchased only with intolerable medical interventions, and ordered that Bouvia be allowed to refuse the feeding tube.

Cruzan v. Director, Missouri Department of Health — The many state courts which have found a right to refuse medical treatment based on a constitutional or common law rationale were joined by the United States Supreme Court in its 1990 decision, <u>Cruzan v. Director, Missouri Department of Health</u>. The case involved Nancy Cruzan, a young woman who had been left by an automobile accident in PVS, and her family's attempt to terminate the artificial nutrition and hydration being administered to her.

<u>Cruzan</u> dealt extensively with the issue of surrogate decision making and will be discussed in more detail as part of the next section, which addresses that subject. However, as part of its decision, the Court recognized that individuals have a constitutionally protected liberty interest in refusing unwanted medical treatment. Cautious of declaring generally what such an interest precisely meant in the context of refusing life-sustaining medical treatment, the Court assumed that a competent person would have a constitutionally protected right to refuse artificial nutrition and hydration, even if it were lifesaving.

<u>Cruzan</u> reflects the increasing recognition by the law of the importance of individual autonomy with regard to treatment decisions, even if the treatments refused are lifesaving and the patient is not suffering from a terminal condition. In fact, this trend is even leading to greater deference in some courts to individual patient choice when the refusal is based upon religious objections to such generally accepted interventions as transfusions.

The constitutional right to refuse treatment is now clear for patients like Mrs. Candura and Mr. Bartling, competent adults who can personally express their refusal at the time treatment is offered. Frequently, however, medical interventions are performed on patients who are unconscious or who have been rendered incapable of informed decision-making by their disease or medication. Yet these individuals may have expressed preferences concerning their care while they were still acknowledged to be competent.

Since the <u>Quinlan</u> case, most states have enacted legislation which seeks to enable individuals to retain some degree of control over their medical treatment, even in the event of incapacity. Some statutes, called **Natural Death Acts** or **Living Wills Acts**, permit individuals to refuse in advance medical procedures, including life-sustaining procedures, by executing advance medical directives. Health professionals are obliged to respect the prior directive at the time such a procedure is indicated, even if the patient has become incompetent in the interval.

The procedures authorized by such statues have proven to be of limited value. Many of the laws require the patient to be diagnosed with a terminal condition in order for the patient's directive to be binding. Other statutes have excluded certain procedures, such as artificial nutrition and hydration, from those which the patient can refuse in advance. In addition, advance refusal of interventions does not allow treatment decisions to be made in light of the particular circumstances which exist at the time a decision is required.

In light of this, many legislatures have passed laws authorizing the use of healthcare surrogates, as another form of decision-making. Called **Durable Power of Attorney for Health Care Acts** or **Health Care Proxy Acts,** these statutes permit one individual to appoint another person to make healthcare decisions by executing a power of attorney or proxy. In the event the person signing such a document becomes incapable of medical decision-making for whatever reason, health professionals can and must then look to the proxy holder as the decision-maker. Such an arrangement permits the individual to choose whatever person is best able to reflect his or her own views and values. A surrogate appointed under proxy or durable power of attorney legislation need not be a family member. The crucial factor is the surrogate's knowledge and respect for the treatment preferences of the one who selected him or her.

In addition to the types of legislation described above, other statutes can create a surrogacy relationship. Every state has mechanisms whereby a guardian or conservator can be appointed for one who is incompetent. The powers of a guardian or conservator may extend to making healthcare decisions for the incompetent ward, provided the ward's condition makes that appropriate. The <u>Quinlan</u> case arose, for example, when Mr. Quinlan asked the court to appoint him Karen's guardian with the authority to order her removed from ventilator support.

The statutes described so far have drawbacks. First, the terms and requirements of the statutes are somewhat technical and may be difficult for some people to understand. Second, many people do not feel comfortable addressing the possibility they might need a surrogate because of what that implies about their vulnerability to illness or injury. The process of having a court appoint a guardian or conservator after an individual is incompetent takes time and money.

Barber v. Superior Court — Courts have recognized that statutory procedures do not provide the exclusive ways for someone to be recognized as another's surrogate. In <u>Barber v. Superior Court,</u> a California appeals court was presented with a situation in which nutrition and hydration had been withdrawn from Clarence Herbert, then in PVS, at the request of his family.

Mr. Herbert had not executed any medical directive, and no guardian or conservator had been appointed. No court reviewed the decision to withdraw treatment prior to Mr. Herbert's death. The physicians who complied with the family's request were subsequently charged with murder. The court of appeals dismissed the charges when it found that the facts presented did not justify criminal charges.

Although the prosecution argued that the family did not have the authority to make treatment decisions in the absence of a formal designation of surrogacy, the court rejected this argument. The court held that the law did not require statutory requirements to be followed in order for the immediate family to make treatment decisions for Mr. Herbert.

Mr. Herbert's wife was the proper person to act as surrogate for her husband, the court ruled. While the surrogate ought to be guided by the patient's own feelings concerning treatment, no prior judicial approval of the surrogate or the surrogate's decision was necessary, in the absence of intrafamily disagreement or evidence of self interest. Therefore the physicians were correct in complying with Mrs. Herbert's request.

Brophy v. New England Sinai Hospital — Other state courts also have concluded that a surrogate's expression of an incompetent patient's wishes should be respected. <u>Brophy v. New England Sinai Hospital</u> involved a 45-year-old who was in PVS as a result of a brain aneurysm. His wife and legal guardian requested the termination of her husband's artificial nutrition, and the attending physician and hospital refused. Massachusetts' highest court ruled that

Mrs. Brophy's request was consistent with a number of statements previously made by her husband about conditions under which he would not want to be kept alive, even though none of the statements specifically mentioned artificial feeding. The court found none of the possible state interests outweighed Mr. Brophy's right to determine the minimum quality of life that made continued treatment worthwhile. As to the state's interest in maintaining medical integrity, the court found that withholding further artificial nutrition was sound medical practice under the circumstances.

In re Jobes — The New Jersey Supreme Court has also concluded that those who best understand the patient's medical attitudes and general value system are best qualified to make substituted judgments for the patient. In re Jobes arose out of a family's request to remove the jejunostomy tube used for feeding a 24-year-old woman who had been in PVS for five years following an unsuccessful surgery. The nursing home in which Jobes was being cared for refused the family's request, and the family sought a court order. The court observed that usually the family of a patient is most concerned with the patient's welfare and is best able to make decisions which are consistent with the patient's wishes. Only if health professionals caring for the patient question the family's ability to protect the patient's interests is a judicially-appointed guardian necessary.

The majority of states which have addressed surrogate decision-making do not require judicial approval of the decisions, as a matter of course. So long as there is no reason to suspect that the surrogate is acting in a manner inconsistent with the patient's wishes, no court intervention is necessary.

A few states, however, have taken the position that a surrogate's decision to withdraw or withhold treatment needs prior judicial approval. For example, Missouri's Supreme Court required in the case of Nancy Cruzan that her parents demonstrate by "clear and convincing" evidence Nancy's explicitly expressed wishes before their order to discontinue Nancy's nutrition would be honored. On appeal, the United States Supreme Court held that Missouri's requirement did not violate Nancy's constitutionally protected rights; each state could decide how best to ensure that a surrogate's decision *for* a patient was the same as that which would be made *by* the patient, were the patient competent to decide.

Missouri's requirement has been widely criticized on a number of grounds. It inserts government into what is essentially a personal sphere. In addition, Missouri's "clear and convincing" standard, combined with the exclusion of certain evidence of Nancy's wishes, seemed designed more to reduce her opportunity to refuse life support than it was designed to ensure accurate surrogate decision-making by her parents. Missouri is one of less than one half-dozen states that require *clear and convincing evidence* of a patient's expressed wishes as a condition of honoring a surrogate's decision to withdraw treatment.

In re Dinnerstein — To date, only one appellate court has considered DNR orders; the Appeals Court of Massachusetts considered the question of the legal authorization of do not resuscitate orders (DNRs) in the 1978 case of <u>In re Dinnerstein</u>. Mrs. Dinnerstein was suffering from advanced Alzheimer's Disease and serious arteriosclerosis. She was paralyzed on one side following a massive stroke, and was "in an essentially vegetative state." Her physician and two children all felt that resuscitation should not be attempted should the patient experience cardiac or respiratory arrest, and they sought to clarify whether prior court approval of such a DNR was required. The court held that no prior court approval was necessary to withhold a treatment alternative (like CPR) which merely suspended the act of dying and could not reasonably be expected to lead to some cure of or relief from the condition being treated.

Artificial Nutrition and Hydration

Artificial nutrition and hydration are medical treatments and can be refused just as any other medical treatment.

Some have argued that a distinction should be made between medical interventions such as respirators and antibiotics, for which refusal should be permitted, and artificial nutrition and hydration, for which refusal should not be permitted. The distinction has been based upon the psychological symbolism of providing food and water to those unable to do so for themselves and upon the inevitability of death in the absence of nutrition and hydration. The natural death and surrogacy statutes of some states, which address artificial nutrition and hydration separately from other treatments, illustrate the continuing vitality of these views.

Appealing though the distinction may initially appear to some, it has not stood up to analysis. The court in <u>Barber v. Superior Court</u> observed that artificial nutrition and hydration were much more similar to other medical procedures than they were to typical human ways of providing food and water, and so their benefits and burdens should be evaluated as any other intervention. The New Jersey Supreme Court in <u>In re Conroy</u>, and the Illinois Supreme Court in <u>In re Estate of Longeway,</u> are only some of the courts which have reached the same conclusion as the <u>Barber</u> court.

The U. S. Supreme Court in <u>Cruzan</u> likewise drew no distinction between nutrition and hydration and other medical procedures. After noting a number of prior state court opinions which rejected any such distinction, the high court assumed that a competent person has a constitutionally protected right to refuse lifesaving nutrition and hydration. This portion of the <u>Cruzan</u> opinion has drawn into question the constitutionality of those state statutes which seek to forbid or make unduly difficult the withdrawal of artificial nutrition and hydration. Such treatments in the future should be evaluated just as any other medical treatment — by assessing the patient's view of their benefits and burdens. ☐

Suggested Readings

• P.S. Applebaum, C.W. Lidz, and A. Meisel, **Informed Consent: Legal Theory and Clinical Practice**. Oxford University Press, 1987.

• Judith Areen, Patricia A. King, Steven Goldberg and Alexander Morgan, **Law, Science and Medicine**. University Casebook Series, 1984.

• Tom Beauchamp and James Childress, **A History and Theory of Informed Consent**. Oxford University Press, 1986.

• A. Edward Doudera and J. Douglas Peters, **Legal and Ethical Aspects of Treating Critically and Terminally Ill Patients**. Aupha Press, 1982.

• The Hastings Center, **Guidelines on the Termination of Life Sustaining Treatment and the Care of the Dying**. The Center, 1987.

• Joanne Lynn, ed., **By No Extraordinary Means: The Choice To Forgo Life Sustaining Food and Water**. Indiana University Press, 1986.

• **Defining Death**. President's Commission for the Study of Ethical Problems in Medicine and Biomedical and Behavior Research, U.S. Government Printing Office, 1981.

• **Deciding to Forgo Life Sustaining Treatment**. President's Commission for the Study of Ethical Problems in Medicine and Biomedical and Behavior Research, U.S. Government Printing Office, 1983.

• James Rachels, **The End of Life**. Oxford University Press, 1986.

• Paul Ramsey, **Ethics at the Edges of Life**. Yale University Press, 1980.

• Tom Regan, **Matters of Life and Death: New Introductory Essays in Moral Philosophy**, 2nd ed. Random House, 1986.

• David H. Smith and Robert M. Veatch, eds., **Guidelines on the Termination of Life-Sustaining Treatment and the Care of the Dying**. Indiana University Press, 1987.

• **The Physician and the Hopelessly Ill Patient: Legal, Medical and Ethical Guidelines**. Society for the Right to Die, 1985.

• Robert M. Veatch, **Death, Dying, and the Biological Revolution; Our Last Quest for Responsibility**. Yale University Press, 1989.

DEVELOPMENT

Developmental and Gender

*It's this very
capacity for devel-
opment within a
structure that lies
at the heart of the
dilemmas the IEC
will encounter....*

T he importance to an IEC of what we call a developmental perspective cannot be overemphasized. As organisms, we are endowed by nature with a capacity for adaptive change, and somewhat paradoxically, change within specific cognitive structures. It's this very capacity for development within a structure that lies at the heart of the dilemmas the IEC will encounter, and at the heart of the process the IEC will engage to resolve those dilemmas.

We receive information from the world and about the world, and at times that information comes into conflict with the organized structure of principles by which we all live our lives. We experience a "jolt," a disjunction or conflict between our structured understanding of the world and the situation presented by reality.

When this occurs, when the "cookbook" no longer works, we're faced suddenly with a range of options, and it's not immediately clear what we ought to do. So we try to adapt. The physician, for example, by principle obligated to preserve life, is confronted with a patient who wants to be disconnected from life support; the physician respects the patient's autonomy, but must also respect her or his own principles. How does the physician simultaneously accommodate the patient's wishes and those principles? How does the physician adapt to a conflicting environment?

*...the process of
ethical delibera-
tion is at heart a
process of
adaptation....*

The IEC deliberation guides and facilitates that adaptive process; the process of ethical deliberation is at heart a process of adaptation, of resolving the basic tensions that develop between the structure of one's principles and the demands of the differing values and principles of patients, families and other professionals.

To help the various actors in an ethical dilemma work effectively through this adaptive process, however, the IEC itself needs a "developmental perspective," a familiarity

DIFFERENCES IN ETHICAL THINKING

with the various stages of ethical development, and with techniques for working with a variety of individuals operating at different levels of development.

Developmental theory sees the human organism as capable of accommodative response to environmental change, yet internally organized within a structure, both physical and cognitive, which is the result of the natural dictates of maturation. Jean Piaget notes the fundamental paradox in this scheme: a living organism is an organized structure that is flexible and open-ended. In a real sense, developmental theory does not resolve the "nature vs. nurture" problems, but rather assimilates both aspects: the human organism is both consistently and internally organized and capable of orderly, adaptive change over time. The developmental perspective understands that the human organism is indeed in a constant state of physical and mental change and transformation.

Complicating the picture is the fact that we never entirely leave behind the "baggage" of earlier stages when moving on to "higher" levels. Rather, the higher levels of functioning generally "inhibit" the lower levels but can be peeled away by stress, exhaustion, intoxication, and certainly by disease. From day to day, even from hour to hour, each of us "slides" up and down the various levels depending on the situation, and in the health care setting, where stresses are particularly high, we're likely to encounter individuals operating at all levels of intellectual and moral functioning.

Consider, for example, the "common cold" of ethical dilemmas, the elderly patient in an ICU in a persistent vegetative state. She has several grown children, all with an interest in her welfare. Because she's in an ICU, there are several physicians consulting on the case, in addition to the

The developmental perspective understands that the human organism is indeed in a constant state of physical and mental change and transformation.

attending physician. There are also a number of nurses from shifts around the clock who are intimately involved in her care, and thus vitally concerned about the disposition of the patient's case.

The patient has created a Durable Power of Attorney for Health Care, and assigned her eldest son as a surrogate decision-maker. But she hasn't given the son any direction as to what she might want in terms of care, or limits on care. The son goes to the IEC and says he wants help thinking the matter through. The attending physician comes to the IEC and says he'll accede to the son's wishes for deliberation by the committee, but that he's learned how to handle cases like this one and doesn't really need the committee's help, except to inform him of the law in this matter.

The physician and the son are operating at two quite different levels of ethical development, and in this case, the son is operating at a more mature level. If someone mentions "potential lawsuit" in this situation — perhaps one of the patient's grown children, or a hospital risk manager — suddenly all the players will be operating at still other, quite disparate levels of ethical reasoning, levels in which fear and outrage may be the dominent emotions.

It's the IEC's job to first recognize how the various players in a particular ethical dilemma may differ in terms of ethical functioning, to respond to each in a way appropriate to that level, and then to work with each of them hopefully to help them move to a more mature level of ethical thinking. It can be difficult, if not futile, for IEC members to communicate in terms of lofty bioethical principles to a physician facing the threat of a lawsuit. Likewise it's just as difficult, if not futile, for the IEC members to talk in terms of concrete medical options with a dying patient's family in need, more than anything else, of human contact.

Recognizing where the actors in an ethical dilemma are operating, and how to communicate effectively with different actors functioning at different levels is a skill that no other ethics committee handbooks discuss. Our intent in this section is to provide the IEC with information to help committee members develop the tools necessary to work with individuals operating at divergent levels of ethical functioning to resolve the dilemma, and at the same time to help them all move to more adaptive levels of ethical functioning.

The Stages of Ethical Development — William Perry's Scheme:

William Perry's research into adult ethical development provides an excellent starting point for IECs to understand and work effectively with individuals operating at varying levels of ethical development.

Perry divides the stages of adult ethical development into three broad positions. In his book, Forms of Intellectual and Ethical Development in the College Years (Holt, Rinehart and Winston, 1968), Perry describes a developmental sequence from strict, simplistic moral dualism to functional relativism and, eventually, to mature commitment.

Perry's research was conducted at Harvard and Radcliffe; his subjects were undergraduates at these schools. He followed these men and women through their careers at the University, and through a series of intensive interviews with them charted changes in their thinking about right and wrong. From these interviews, he identified the three broad positions, with gradations within each position, as typical

Perry divides the stages of adult ethical development into three broad positions...

of the stages through which we all develop.

However, as noted above, these stages are "situational," that is, our level of ethical functioning depends on the context in which we're operating, and on our familiarity with the context. Thus a relative of a dying patient, new to the healthcare setting, will likely operate at the earliest, very naive stage of ethical reasoning when dealing with that patient's physicians, while he or she may operate at more mature levels within the context of his or her own career or personal life.

With time and experience in the clinical setting, however, that individual may move "up" the developmental hierarchy, at least in terms of his or her dealings in the clinical setting. Likewise, healthcare professionals, "at home" in this clincial setting, may normally operate at a higher level of ethical reasoning, but under stress, when fatigued or, as noted above, when stressed by such things as the threat of a suit, may slide "down" the scale.

It's important that the IEC understand the possibilty for movement through the positions, and when possible help the actors in an ethical dilemma make those developmental leaps. It's also important that the IEC understand what Perry calls "detours" or "roadblocks" in the individual's development from one stage to the next. These detours will be of particular interest to IECs since they'll inevitably encounter men and women blocked in the developmental process, and who can cause the committee a variety of problems.

Position One — Moral Dualism: People operating at this level or position are authority-oriented. For them, obedience to authority is the valued virtue or way of behaving. They tend to see the world as a dualism, in terms of we/

right/good versus other/wrong/bad. For them, right answers exsit in the absolute, and they believe these answers are known to an authority who possesses and can disclose the answers.

An ethical dilemma is experienced by those operating at this level as a question of right or wrong. They tend not to understand that an ethical dilemma is in fact a conflict between goods or values, and that other well-meaning individuals can legitimately hold opposing views. They'll tend to perceive principles as rules; when they encounter an ethical dilemma, the question for them is how to make the applicable rules work in this particular case.

This isn't to say these individuals aren't compassionate, of course. Rather, their compassion can be bounded by principles which they perceive, sometimes incorrectly, as rules. For example, in the case of a dying patient who asks that food and nutrition be withdrawn, or whose family makes the request, the authority-oriented healthcare professional may assume there are rules, religious prohibitions or even laws against such withdrawal. Intuitively, they may know that withdrawal is in the patient's best interest, but they'll feel hemmed in by the "law," so they'll come to the IEC asking the IEC to say this action is OK or it's not. They'll come wanting clarity about the rule.

The IEC will recognize individuals operating at this level by the questions they ask when they come to the committee. In general, their language and attitude toward the IEC will be indicative of a perception of the IEC as the authority; their questions will tend to involve answers to dilemmas; individuals operating at this level will talk about the IEC in "authoritative" terms.

Individuals operating at this authority-oriented level will tend to view those who don't agree with them as wrong, and thus they can present a challenge to the quality of IEC deliberations, since such deliberations are a forum which depends, for effectiveness, on the presumed good will of all those involved.

Thus the IEC needs to be very sensitive to the needs and expectations of those operating at this level. Since the committee works specifically as a forum to resolve conflicts of value, authority-oriented individuals seeking specific and authoritative answers will be very uncomfortable with the deliberative process. If they come to the committee and give the clear message that they do want an answer from some authority, they should perhaps not be involved in committee deliberations. Rather, the IEC should invite them to provide information, thank them for coming, and tell them: "We'll have our discussion now, and let you know in an hour or so what we talked about."

The committee should not relate the entire content of the discussion, in "raw" form with all its expressed uncertainties and doubts, to the individual operating at this level. Rather, the committee should give that person specific, tightly focused recommendations.

Also, those operating at this level tend to have a strong law-orientation, since the law in their minds is definitive (any good lawyer will tell you that's not at all the case), thus it's a very good idea, when presenting a recommendation to someone operating at this level, especially to a physician, to be very specific about applicable case law, and whatever statutory law applies to the case under consideration.

The Transition From the First to Second Position: While we think of individuals operating in the first position as "naive" in terms of ethical thinking, in truth it's not at all unusual for physicians to operate in the authority-oriented realm, since all their training has been presented from an authority-oriented position and many have internalized that to become the authority.

As mentioned above, families encountering the healthcare system for the first time likely will invest that physician with an absolute authority to determine answers to clinical problems, and for the physician operating in this authority-oriented position as well, the relationship is comfortable, and even rewarding.

But in the modern clinical environment, where a variety of medical specialists may be called in to consult on a single, seriously ill patient's case, the naive family of that patient will inevitably begin to hear a number of specialists, all with narrow and well-defined areas of expertise, differing, sometimes wildly, on diagnosis, treatment plans and prognoses.

While the family came to the medical experts for authoritative answers, now the family finds itself confronted by a seeming chaos of uncertainties. It's a difficult, painful period for the family, and yet the experts' uncertainties and the seeming chaos of the modern clinical environment may well stimulate the family's development from the authority-oriented position to a more mature level of ethical reasoning.

It's a process of development identical to that which Perry observed in college students; they come to the University expecting answers, and instead must begin to confront the uncertainties of the experts from whom they'd originally sought those answers; this hopefully sparks the beginning of more complex and sophisticated ways of thinking about what is right or wrong.

In Perry's study, however, college students typically took 18 months to two years to make the transition from an authority-oriented position to the relativistic stage. In the clinical setting, we've seen adults encountering a barrage of opinions from a variety of authority figures lose their basic belief and trust in authority in a matter of days or weeks. And as they lose their foundation — that sense of being anchored, which is provided by an authority-oriented position — they can become confused, and out of that confusion comes frustration, a certain combativeness, and even anger.

Physicians or other caregivers confronted by angry family members at this stage may not realize that the family's aggressiveness or combativeness is actually a sign of maturation; caregivers can become defensive in the face of this process, and communication often breaks down.

While this aggressiveness is a symptom of maturation, this is no consolation for the family members going through the process, or for the healthcare professionals who may be the focus of that anger and frustration. When a case ends up before the IEC in which such tensions figure, it's important that the IEC validate the concerns of of the family members and try to "calm the waters," otherwise a good discussion will be difficult.

By recognizing when individuals are operating at this level, or when individuals are in the process of transition, and by presenting material that is most accessible to that level, the IEC can meet the needs of those involved in the dilemma and also gently help them along the path to a more mature level of ethical reasoning.

In particular, the information gathering portion of the methodology can be particularly helpful at this point. If the IEC co-chairs carefully evoke from the consulting physicians, and primary care physician and nurses a consensus about the actual prognosis of the patient. The prognosis is an important unifying element in any clinical situation, and coming to consensus about the prognosis can help bring forth a more "holistic" picture of the situation for both the patient's family and the caregivers, easing some of the tensions and frustrations that can arise from conflicting or divergent opinions about probable outcomes.

The IEC should also be aware that family members or even staff members at this transitional stage in which faith in previous authorities has been shaken, may come to the IEC expecting the committee itself to take the place of the previous authority figures. In this case, the IEC needs to carefully work with those involved to help them understand the probabilistic nature of any prognosis.

The Second Position — Relativism: When the naive trust in authority disolves, the individuals begin — hopefully — to acknowledge the fact that people of good will can and will differ in their values and beliefs, and that this doesn't mean those who differ are "good" or "bad."

At the earliest levels of this position — a level of absolute relativism — the attitude might be expressed as: "Your guess is as good as mine." With somewhat more maturity, however, persons in this position modify their thinking to a realization that we work in a society of individual diversity, and for society to function, we have to agree on general norms. These norms are relative and certainly not derived from authority, but rather, as a matter of convenience, serve to accomplish limited goals.

Rules thus become very important for people at this position, not rules out of authority, but rules of process, rules for fair play, for "working things out." Procedural rules create a setting in which all the players view themselves as equal, in which compromises can be made, but in which there's no longer the expectation of "right" answers. The virtues valued by those operating at this position are fair play, the ability to compromise, tolerance, and respect for differences.

Individuals who enter into the process of ethical deliberation from this position often have had experience in the healthcare setting before, and thus have already experienced the sort of dislocation that results in the movement from the authority-oriented position to a relativistic position. Once an individual has reached this level in his or her experience with healthcare, there's no going back. The individual will never believe in the absolute authority of medical experts again.

An individual operating at this level may come to the IEC saying, "I'm really stymied by this problem and I'd like to have a process of discussion or reflection to work out a compromise we can all live with, some sort of ad hoc consensus about this question." It's a fundamentally different position from the first, and the IEC can safely include these individuals in the deliberative process itself, and indeed, these individuals probably would expect to be part of the deliberative process.

The maturest level of this position acknowledges that each expert has expertise in certain areas, but does not at all accept the idea that that expertise can be generalized into other areas; this position will defer to the expert in that expert's specific area of competence, but will expect the expert to function as a member of a team in other areas.

The Third Position — Evolving Commitments: Individuals operating at this level have, in Perry's scheme, developed from relativism to what he calls commitment. But commitment to what?

Perry relates Commitment to an "affirmatory experience" through which we continuously define our identity
and involvements in the world. Commitments, he continues, refer to affirmations and require the courage of responsibility and presuppose "an acceptance of human limita-
tions, including the limits of reason".

The primary virtue for those operating at this level is not
obedience, nor fair play and negotiation, but integrity, and
specifically that integrity which derives from acting consistently with an internalized set of principles. Authority, for
those operating in position three, comes from within.
Negotiation, for such a person, is not an issue; he or she will
act in accordance only with those internalized principles.

At first glance, such an invidual would seem to present
the IEC with enormous problems. For the individual operating at the principled level, whatever act is in keeping with
his or her own principles is right. Certainly such an individual is not interested in whatever "authorities" have to say
on the matter, nor is such an individual interested in getting
others to adhere to his or her principles.

The dying woman who decides to forgo therapies to die
at home, who says "I've made up my mind" to physicians
or relatives who plead with her to continue treatment may
be operating at the principled level. Such an individual is no
longer concerned with what the "authorities" say, whether
that authority comes in the form of a medical expert, or case
or statutory law. She'll pose possible dilemmas for the
caregivers or family, but there is certainly no dilemma here
from her standpoint.

The litmus test of this position is adherence to principles
even when this means a negative outcome; Gandhi and
Martin Luther King are classic examples of individuals
willing to face jail and even death for strongly held prin-

ciples. Such individuals are quite capable of operating at the other two levels, however, if need be; they can act as authorities, or abide by the decisions of authorities, or enter into negotiations with others and make compromises, to a point, and that point is always reached when the issue involves their own integrity. Thus the dying woman mentioned above might well abide by the medical expert's advice concerning treatment to make her comfortable at home. She might well negotiate and compromise in terms of care options, as long as those options are completely in accordance with her decision to die at home.

This isn't to say that the person operating at this level is free of ambiguities, dilemmas or confusion; after all, how does such a person know the principles by which she has chosen to act, despite the consequences, are the right principles? It's a fundamental question anyone operating at this level will constantly be asking; it's a fundamental question in philosophy: are there objective, external norms by which we know a principled act is the right act?

This, then, takes us full circle, back to the fundamental question of ethics, but in truth, the IEC will only rarely encounter such individuals in a clinical setting. Of more immediate concern to IEC members are those who've made what Perry refers to as "detours" in their ethical development. These individuals will cause the IEC no end of headaches.

Detours: As Perry's development scheme has been presented here, the implication is that we all progress steadily from one position to the next. In fact, the line of development is hardly steady, nor always in one direction; rather, we sometimes stall, sometimes escape from development entirely, and sometimes reverse direction.

As noted above, the transition from the first, authority-oriented position to the second, relativistic position, can be extremely painful when the "authority" on which we relied for "truth" proves fallible and we find ourselves confronting the vast, anarchic realm of "moral relativism." We described above the problems a person going through this transition can face, particularly in the clinical setting. But what happens when the individual confronts "moral relativism" and then doesn't make the transition?

Perry identifies three possible roadblocks or detours at this point. They are temporizing, escape into addictive behavior, and retreat to an "authoritarian" postion.

Temporizing: When we temporize, we simply refuse to move from one position to the next. In the clinical setting, temporizing is most often evident in those who refuse to move within the relativism position from absolute relativism to a more sophisticated level in which they come to recognize the need for negotiation and compromise. They'll say "What I do is as good as what you do, so let's stay out of one another's way and do our own things."

When encountering such an individual, perhaps the most effective strategy for the IEC is to invite the person to attend to some of the evidence that "it's not quite so simple," that his or her choices do affect others.

Escape: It's not at all surprising that we see a high incidence of drug and alcohol addiction in the health professions. Addiction can provide an escape for some from what they perceive as the chaos of relativism.

But a much more common form of addicition the IEC will encounter in its dealings with healthcare professionals is "work-aholism," and it's usually the primary care physician or primary care nurse who says "I don't have time for this philosophical nonsense; I have patients to care for, lives

temporizing

escape

"work-aholism"

to save." What they're really saying is they don't have time to deal with basic issues of human values because they're afraid to confront these issues. And not only are they afraid to confront these issues, they lack the skills for managing compromises when faced with those with competing values.

How do you deal with this? Politely, but firmly explain to the person: "There are others who do have concerns and who must work through the process, and your participation in the process would be extremely helpful."

Retreat to an Authoritarian Position: In confronting relativism, some retreat to an authoritarian position. This is by far the most troublesome "detour" the IEC will encounter and please note that in Perry's scheme there's a very clear distinction between the first position — the "authority-oriented" position — and the detour to an authoritarian position.

The person operating at the authority-oriented level will be looking for someone to provide answers. This person is very interested in finding out what the experts say he or she should do. Conversely, the person who has retreated to the authoritarian position will expect everyone else to obey authority; they'll even demand that authority itself follow what is perceived to be "objective" law. In the clinical setting, such individuals occasionally will take troubling cases to the police, to the press, or, in cases involving children, to child protective agencies. If they come to the IEC, they'll come not for reflection, but demanding that the IEC act as a "policing" agency to force others to obey whatever standards they believe should be adhered to.

These individuals are in a process of regression. Faced with relativism, they've pulled back, and are trying to control the external environment so it won't give them messages they don't want to hear. They may view the IEC and the work it does as a direct threat to whatever "authority" provides them with "truth." Thus they may tend to work against the new IEC, especially when the IEC is starting its work.

In our experience, in a hospital, nursing home, hospice or other healthcare institution with a large staff, it's almost certain at least one member of the staff will be in this state of regresssion. Somewhat paradoxically, such individuals have retreated to the authoritarian position precisely because they don't believe that authority has the answers; they're trying to recreate a stable world through a construct, and deep down they know it's a construct. Thus moving them beyond that construct is very, very difficult.

It's very difficult for the IEC to do anything about such individuals; the only way to get them back on the track of ethical development is first to resolve their anxieties, which is beyond the purview of IECs. In dealing with such individuals, the IEC needs to be carefully accurate about the boundaries of the law, so they understand that whatever recommendations it makes, it is within the boundaries such individuals will recognize.

Gender Differences:

It's a fact of life that, like it or not, most physicians are men and most nurses are women. This is changing, of course, but slowly, and the present reality has important implications for IECs — there are fundamental gender differences in the way men and women process ethical questions, as well as developmental differences.

In our discussions above, we relied heavily on Perry's researches, which did not tap gender differences. To the extent women develop differently, these differences were seen by developmental theorists as a problem in women's development; "different" was seen as better or, in the case of ethical development in women, worse. Freud says: "for women the level of what is ethically normal is different from what it is in men."

Freud concluded that "women show less sense of justice than men, that they are less ready to submit to the great exigencies of life, that they are more often influenced in their judgements by feelings of affection or hostility."

In her book on gender differences in moral development, *In A Different Voice*, Carol Gilligan suggests that the "failure of women to fit existing models of human growth may point to a problem in the representation, a limitation in the conception of human condition, an omission of certain truths about life." She says Freud and the others are quite right, women are different, and thank God for that. Freud's error, like that of others, was assuming that this difference resulted from some aberrant or stunted development.

What Freud saw as a weakness in women's moral development — "they are too often influenced by feelings" — is from Gilligan's perspective a strength. The masculine perspective underlying all discussions of ethical development presuppose a world of separate individuals; in the established scheme of masculine ethical development, the basic social interaction is competition for affection, goods, status, achievement, everything. The highest level of ethical development occurs when the concept of justice is embraced, and for those (men) operating at this level, the challenge is to equalize the playing field and give everyone an equal opportunity to compete on an equal basis. Affirmative action and equal opportunity laws derive directly from this perspective.

From the feminine perspective, the important issue is not justice, but relationship. Jean Piaget noted this in his study of rules and respect for rules. Girls, he noted, had a more relaxed attitude about rules; they were willing to make exceptions, which boys weren't; while little boys would argue endlessly about the rules, little girls were more reconciled to innovation. As a result, the "legal sense" which Piaget thought essential to moral development was "far less developed in little girls."

But while Piaget saw this lack of a "legal sense" as a flaw, Gilligan celebrates the lack (and considering the cost of our litigiousness, perhaps we all should). When disputes about rules developed, girls were much more likely to quit the game, Piaget noted, and Gilligan expands on this fact: for the girls, relationships were more valuable than competition.

Rather than "level the playing field" and allow everyone to compete on an equal basis, women strive for the establishment and preservation of relationships. Rather than emphasis on a "level playing field," the feminine perspective takes into account individual differences and the fact that some need more than others, then tries to find a way to accommodate those differences.

This difference in perspective can be seen in the clinical setting: the husband or son or male physician will say let's give the patient "every possible chance," a sentiment that derives directly from the masculine perspective of justice. The nursing staff, in the same situation, will frequently say: "Look what this is doing to the family." Or they may say: "Look at what this is doing to my unit." They see the patient as embedded in the family system, or in a larger system within the nursing unit. They see the patient in the context of relationship.

For the IEC, it's important to understand these two perspectives, and try to build some rapprochement between the differing perspectives. One perspective is not more valuable than another; both perspectives exist in the human mind, in men and women alike; it's not a matter of replacing one with the other, but of learning to appreciate and understand both perspectives. □

Suggested Readings

• Ronald Duska and Mariellen Whelan, **Moral Development, A Guide to Piaget and Kohlberg.** Paulist Press, 1975.

* Carol Gilligan, **In a Different Voice**, second ed. Harvard University Press, 1986.

• William G. Perry, Jr., **Forms of Intellectual and Ethical Development in the College Years.** Holt, Rinehart and Winston, Inc., 1968.

APPENDICES

COMMITTEE EDUCATION

W e strongly recommend that the IEC establish an education subcommittee to serve a variety of functions, beginning with intensive didactic instruction for committee members initially, and continuing thereafter with regular educational programs for the committee as a whole, as well as for hospital staff and the community at large.

At the Outset: All committee members should receive formal, organized education by experts in four areas: (1) ethical theory and the history of ethics with a focus on medical ethics; (2) legal issues, how the law works, how decisions are made and the real implications of precedential cases; (3) process education, that is, how to do a case consultation, how the methodology is applied and the possible pitfalls in the clinical environment, some psychological theory and practical information about the impact of illness and grieving; and (4) how to run a successful meeting.

This manual is intended to form a foundation and provide a resource for such instruction, but we also feel the manual will be most useful used in conjunction with experts brought in to instruct the committee members in the specific areas outlined above and with additional instructional materials from the listings included in the previous chapters.

Ongoing IEC Education: The subcommittee should be responsible for establishing, maintaining and expanding a library of books, articles, journals and audiovisual materials relevant to committee functioning. The subcommittee should also be responsible for reviewing and analyzing key articles on specific issues for other committee members, and presenting packages of such materials at each meeting. In a sense, the education subcommittee can also function as the archivist for the IEC, collecting and organizing reports from case consultations, and making them available for new members.

The education subcommittee should also consider doing retrospective case reviews; this provides a "debriefing" for those members involved in the case, and allows them to consider what pitfalls they encountered, and reflect on what they've learned.

Finally, education subcommittee members should attend special topic conferences locally and nationally themselves, as well as seek out experts both locally and nationally and arrange for them to come to speak to the IEC.

Institutional Education: In a sense, the education subcommittee functions as the IEC's "public relations arm." By providing educational opportunities for the hospital staff about ethical issues, the education subcommittee will educate the staff about the IEC itself, what it does and how it functions.

Hospital education should be approached developmentally, beginning with ethics grand rounds or presentations to the medical staff by experts from outside. Next, as the IEC develops experience and confidence, its members should begin to give presentations themselves. Finally, we strongly urge IECs to do ethics rounds on a rotating basis in the various clinical units that are likely to refer cases to the IEC. This hones the clinical skills of the committee members at the same time it begins to initiate the medical and nursing staffs into the process of ethical reflection, and educates them in what the IEC has to offer. In our practice on rounds, we generally suggest that IECs structure meetings with the staff of a clinical unit monthly, alternating between a didac-

institutional education

tic presentation on some specific bioethical issue, and an actual case review.

Community Education: The community ought to know the IEC exists, and what its purpose is, and that the community is welcome to refer cases to it. A major component of community education should cover prior directives, since so many of the cases that come before the IEC involve situations in which caregivers are trying to make decisions about the care of unconscious or comatose patients.

This sort of community education, particularly about prior directives and durable powers of attorney, should be done in conjunction with medical staff education, however. The IEC shouldn't "turn a community loose" on the medical staff without also providing the medical staff with all the resources it needs to answer a patient's questions. ☐

Policies And Guidelines

F orming a policy and guidelines subcommittee offers several benefits. First, the hospital community, and particularly the medical staff and the administration, will be seeking some assistance in crafting various policies that are required by the JCAHO, as well as by local and state regulations and laws. The IEC thus is in a position to be the mechanism for fulfilling such regulations, and providing a valuable service to the hospital.

Second, the formation of a policy and guidelines subcommittee, and the activities of that subcommittee, will give the IEC some productive work to do while still learning the process of case consultation; this will give the IEC members a clear sense they are accomplishing important, concrete results even as they learn skills for consultation.

Third, in the process of forming policy and guidelines, the subcommittee will engage the medical and nursing staffs in the process of ethical reflection. The IEC members will enter into dialogue with these staff members about prevalent ethical issues they deal with all the time, sensitizing both themselves and the staff. This will help educate the medical and nursing staffs about the IEC and the process of ethical consultation, and it will allow the IEC members to become better acquainted with the other staff.

In the process of forming policy and guidelines, the subcommittee will engage the medical and nursing staffs in the ethical process.

Policies and Guidelines

Some of the policies and guidelines the IEC will want to consider include:

Informed Consent: While drafting policies regarding informed consent, the IEC can also use policy development as a way to educate the hospital community about the fundamental importance of informed consent.

Some issues embedded in any discussion of informed consent, which the IEC will want to discuss, include competency and capacity, the importance of a medical evaluation and recommendation, surrogacy, and the right of refusal.

Forgoing Therapy: This broad category includes withholding and withdrawing therapy, DNR orders, and nutrition and hydration. Each IEC should have some policies and guidelines developed around these issues, and these policies and guidelines should take into consideration whatever decisions about these matters have been made by local jurisdictions. In particular, there is specific legislation in some states that addresses the issues of nutrition and hydration, and the IEC will want to educate itself and the hospital community about local jurisdictions. Again, the policy development process can become an educational tool in this regard.

Categories of Patients: Another set of policies or guidelines should include categories of patients, rather than actions. Depending on each hospital's patient population, these categories might include neonates, AIDS patients, the frail elderly, rehabilitation patients, patients with chronic, degenerative nerve disorders, and burn victims. This list is not exhaustive; again, each IEC will have to analyze the patient population of its own hospital to determine which patient categories should be covered.

Confidentiality: This is the most neglected of all ethical principles in healthcare, and one that the IEC will hopefully address in policy terms; in so doing, the IEC will help

forgoing therapy

categories of patients

confidentiality

educate and remind the hospital community of the fundamental importance of this principle.

The Nature of Policies and Guidelines

The goal of policy and guideline formation is not so much
to develop exhaustive policies that anticipate every possible contingency, but rather to engage specific hospital
units, to enter into a dialogue about specific ethical issues
with the staff in each of these units, and to educate them
about the IEC and about ethical deliberation. ☐

Evaluation Of The IEC

H ow does the IEC know it's doing a good job? There are several ways to tell, and these can be broken down roughly into external and internal indicators of effectiveness.

Externally: Perhaps the simplest way the IEC can know it's doing an effective job is to ask. Do a survey. In doing so, the IEC can assess not only its performance, but the hospital community's knowledge of ethical issues.

A more subtle external measure of an IEC's effectiveness is the impact the IEC's activities have on litigation. If the IEC is working effectively, there will be fewer requests for the hospital legal counsel to clean up messes, or fewer threats of litigation.

Internally: Internal measures of IEC success include the vitality of what we call a "moral community." Are people willing to say things others are willing to disagree with, and yet all can work together? If so, it's a good sign the IEC is functioning well.

Attendance is a real measure of effectiveness; absences or a high turnover can be indicators the IEC is not being as effective as it could be.

We recommend that the IEC members take at least one retreat, and better yet two, each year. These are usually one-day meetings. The most successful IECs we've seen generally have two each year, one devoted to the didactic review of some specific ethical issue, often with an expert brought in. The second annual retreat is devoted to self- evaluation; members come together to discuss the ethical process as they've practiced it, and to evaluate themselves. Generally speaking, the members of an effective IEC enjoy these retreats, and one another's company, while gradually increasing their competence and confidence levels. ☐

external evaluation

internal evaluation

attendance

JCAHO Guidelines

Note, the following is an excerpt from the Joint Commission 1991 guidelines for institutional accreditation. Healthcare institutions are rated on the basis of implementation of systems for resolving ethical issues.

Intent of Rl.1.1.6 through Rl.1.1.6.1 — Health care professionals provide patient care within an ethical framework established by the profession, the health care organization, and the law. The health care professional has an obligation to respect the voice of the patient, or his/her designated representative, when ethical issues arise during the patient's care. The health care organization has an obligation to incorporate the patient, or his/her designated representative, in the organization's mechanism established to consider such issues.

The organization also has the responsibility to educate staff and care recipients in the ethical issues that arise in health care. Such education may include community programs, inclusion of care recipients in educational programs, and sponsoring education programs on ethical issues for organization and staff members.

Scoring for Rl.1.1.6 — There is a process(es) or mechanism(s) established to include the patient or his/her designated representative in discussions of ethical issues surrounding his/her care. For example, the organization provides access to ethics consultants or an ethics committee, as appropriate.

Scoring for R1.1.1.6.1 — The organization has implemented a mechanism(s) (for example, an ethics committee, ethics forum, consultation services, or a combination of such) to consider and discuss ethical issues arising in patient care. Health care professionals participate in the discussion and resolution of ethical issues and are furnished with the educational resources necessary to assist them in the evaluation of the alternatives available. The mechanism(s) includes a means of educating care recipients in the ethical issues surrounding health care. □

THE DANFORTH AMENDMENT

The Patient Self-Determination Act, sponsored by Senator John C. Danforth (R-Missouri), was included in the Omnibus Budget Reconciliation Act of 1990. Though it passed with little notice, the law, which took effect on December 1, 1991, will likely have a profound impact on healthcare institutions nationwide. It applies not only to hospitals, but to long term care facilities, hospices, home health agencies, HMOs, and a variety of other medical institutions and agencies. The PSDA requires these institutions to inform patients of their right to control decisions regarding their own health care.

Specific sections of the Act require institutions to:

• provide all patients with clear, accurate information regarding their right to make healthcare decisions, existing state laws and regulations which help patients to enact those decisions, and institutional policies and procedures for implementing patients' decisions;

• document in the medical record whether the patient has executed a prior directive such as a "living will" or a Durable Power of Attorney for Healthcare Decisions;

• guarantee that care is not contingent on whether a patient has created a prior directive;

• ensure that state laws and regulations regarding prior directives are followed within institutions;

• offer immunity and staff education programs regarding prior directives and related issues.

Most individuals who create advanced directives try to do

so in the context of a conversation with their primary care physicians. In our experience, we find that most practicing physicians are not adequately prepared for such conversations and defer them indefinitely until the patient is in acute medical crisis and unable to participate in a decision-making process.

Thus we suggest that healthcare institutions create in-depth educational programs to help medical staffs initiate and carry out instructive conversations regarding end-of-life decisions with their patients. While educational efforts can take a variety of forms, we suggest that any program contain three key elements:

Timing: as the PSDA is implemented at the institutional level and more patients become aware of their right to create prior directives, requests to physicians for discussions about choices will increase. Educational programs created for physicians can be prepared in advance, and implemented as medical staff experience a need to learn the skills required for such conversations.

Content: theoretical, long-winded expositions will be ineffective with busy primary care physicians; rather, very clear, concrete, distilled materials focusing on behavioral skills will be of greatest help.

Delivery: while role-playing would be most efficient to convey skills, physicians usually are very reluctant to engage in such self-revealing exercises. We've found that brief didactic presentations, accompanied by good slides, work best, especially when followed by carefully prepared printed materials and instructional video tapes which can be viewed and read at home. ☐

Recommended Resources In Bioethics

Suggested Journals and Newsletters:

American Journal of Law and Medicine
Bioethics
Cambridge Quarterly
Hastings Center Report
HEC Forum
Journal of Medical Ethics (UK)
Journal of Medical Humanities and Bioethics
Journal of Medicine and Philosophy
Law, Medicine and Health Care
Milbank Memorial Fund Quarterly
New Titles in Bioethics (available from
    Kennedy Institute of Ethics)
Second Opinion
Society for Health and Human Values Bulletin
Theoretical Medicine
(Many medical and nursing journals regularly carry articles of importance to IECs. These include the *New England Journal of Medicine*, the *Journal of the American Medical Association*, the *Journal of the American Nursing Association*, and the *Archives of Internal Medicine*.)

Selected Bibliography of Books:

Ethical Theory

• Tom L. Beauchamp, **Philosophical Ethics**. McGraw Hill, 1982.
• Robert N. Bellah, Richard Madsen, William M. Sullivan, Ann Swidler, and Steven M. Tipton, **Habits of the Heart**. University of California Press, 1985.

• Carol Gilligan, **In a Different Voice** (2nd ed.). Harvard University Press, 1983.

• Carol Gilligan, Janie Victoria Ward, Jill McLean Taylor, with Bettie Bardige, **Mapping the Moral Domain**. Harvard University Press, 1988.

• J.L. Mackie, **Ethics: Inventing Right and Wrong**. Penguin Books, Ltd., 1977.

• James Rachels, **The Elements of Moral Philosophy**. Random House, 1986.

Medical Ethics

• Tom L. Beauchamp and James L. Childress, **Principles of Biomedical Ethics** (3rd edition). Oxford University Press, 1989.

• Tom L. Beauchamp and LeRoy Walters, eds., **Contemporary Issues in Bioethics** (3rd edition). Wadsworth Publishing Company, 1989.

• Tom L. Beauchamp and Laurence B. McCullough, **Medical Ethics — the Moral Responsibilities of Physicians**. Prentice-Hall, 1984.

• Baruch A. Brody, **Life and Death Decision Making**. Oxford University Press, 1988.

• Baruch A. Brody and H. Tristram Engelhardt, Jr., **Bioethics: Readings and Cases**. Prentice Hall, 1987.

• Allen E. Buchanan and Dan W. Brock, **Deciding for Others: The Ethics of Surrogate Decision Making**. Cambridge University Press, 1989.

• Ronald J. Christie and C. Barry Hoffmaster, **Ethical Issues in Family Medicine**. Oxford University Press, 1986.

• H. Tristram Engelhardt, **The Foundations of Bioethics**. Oxford University Press, 1986.

• Glenn C. Graber and David C. Thomasma, **Theory and Practice in Medical Ethics**. Continuum Publishing Co., 1989.

• Albert Jonson, Mark Siegler, William J. Winslade, **Clinical Ethics** (2nd ed). Macmillan Publishing Co., 1986.

• Ruth Macklin, **Mortal Choices: Bioethics in Today's World**. Pantheon, 1987.

• Edmund Pellegrino and David C. Thomasma, **For the Patient's Good: The Restoration of Beneficence in Health Care**. Oxford University Press, 1988.

• Paul Ramsey, **The Patient as Person: Explorations in Medical Ethics**. Yale University Press, 1970.

• Warren T. Reich, **The Encyclopedia of Bioethics**. Kennedy

Institute of Ethics, 1982.

• Stanley Joel Reiser, Arthur J. Dyck and William J. Curran, eds., **Ethics in Medicine**. The MIT Press, 1982.

• Margery W. Shaw and A. Edward Doudera, eds., **Defining Human Life**. Aupha Press, 1983.

• Stuart F. Spicker and H. Tristram Engelhardt, Jr., eds., **Philosophical Medical Ethics: Its Nature and Significance**. D. Reidel, 1977.

• Robert M. Veatch, ed., **Cross Cultural Perspectives in Medical Ethics: Readings**. Jones and Bartlett, 1989.

• Robert M. Veatch, **A Theory of Medical Ethics**. Basic Books, 1981.

• LeRoy Walters and Tamar Joy Kahn, **Bibliography of Bioethics**. Kennedy Institute of Ethics, 1975.

• Richard Zaner, **Ethics and the Clinical Encounter**. Prentice Hall, 1988.

Nursing Ethics

• **Nursing: A Social Policy Statment**. American Nurses Association, 1980.

• J. Ashly, **Hospitals, Paternalism, and the Role of the Nurse**. St. Martin's Press, 1976.

• Elsie L. Bandman and Bertram Bandman, **Nursing Ethics in the Life Span**. Appleton-Century Crofts, 1985.

• Martin Benjamin and Joy Curtis, **Ethics in Nursing**. Oxford University Press, 1981.

• J. Q. Benoliel, **The Nurse and the Dying Patient**. Macmillan, 1967.

• A. Carmi and S. Schneider, eds., **Nursing Law and Ethics**. Springer-Verlag, 1985.

• Helen Creighton, **Law Every Nurse Should Know**. W. B. Saunders Company, 1981.

• Leah Curtin and M. Josephine Flaherty, **Nursing Ethics Theories and Pragmatics**. Brady Communications Co., Inc., 1982.

• Kathleen M. Fenner, **Ethics and Law in Nursing**. Van Nostrand Reinhold Company, 1980.

• Janine Fiesta, **The Law and Liability**. John Wiley & Son, 1983.

• Marsha D. M. Fowler and June Levine-Arliff, **Ethics at the Bedside**. J. B. Lippincott Company, 1987.

• Sharol F. Jacobson and H. Marie McGrath, eds., **Nurses Under Stress**. John Wiley & Sons, 1983.

• A. Jameton, **Nursing Practice: The Ethical Issues**. Prentice Hall, 1984.

• T. Pence, **Ethics in Nursing: An Annotated Bibliography**, 2nd ed. National League for Nursing, 1986.

• S. Reverby, **Ordered to Care: The Dilemma of American Nursing**. Cambridge University Press, 1986.

• Karen Brodkin Sacks, **Caring by the Hour**. University of Illinois Press, 1988.

• Ian E. Thompson, Kath M. Melia and Kenneth M. Boyd, **Nursing Ethics**. Churchill Livingston, 1983.

• Joyce E. Thompson and Henry O. Thompson, **Bioethical Decision Making for Nurses**. Appelton-Century Crofts, 1985.

• Robert M. Veatch and Sara T. Fry, **Case Studies in Nursing Ethics**. J. B. Lippincott Company, 1987.

The Professional/Patient Relationship

• Paul S. Appelbaum, W. Charles, and Alan Meisel, **Informed Consent: Legal Theory and Clinical Practice**. Oxford University Press, 1987.

• Sisella Bok, **Lying**. Pantheon Press, 1978.

• Eric Cassell, **The Healer's Art**. MIT Press, 198.

• James F. Childress, **Who Should Decide? Paternalism in Health Care**. Oxford University Press, 1982.

• Ruth Faden and Tom L. Beuchamp, **A History and Theory of Informed Consent**. Oxford University Press, 1986.

• Jay Katz, **The Silent World of Doctor and Patient**. Macmillan Press, 1984.

• William May, **The Physician's Covenant**. Westminster Press, 1983.

• **Making Health Care Decisions**, President's Commission for the Study of Ethical Problems in Medicine and Biomedical and Behavioral Research. U.S. Government Printing Office, 1982-83.

Withdrawal of Treatment/Death and Dying

• A. Edward Doudera and J. Douglas Peters, **Legal and Ethical Aspects of Treating Critically and Terminally Ill Patients**. Aupha Press, 1982.

• The Hastings Center, **Guidelines on the Termination of Life Sustaining Treatment and the Care of the Dying**. The Center, 1987.

• Joanne Lynn, ed., **By No Extraordinary Means: The Choice To**

Forgo Life Sustaining Food and Water. Indiana University Press, 1986.

• John C. Moskop and Loretta Kopelman, **Ethics and Critical Care Medicine**. D. Reidel, 1985.

• **Institutional Protocols for Decisions About Life Sustaining Treatments: A Special Report**. Office of Technology Assessment, U.S. Government Printing Office, 1988.

• **Defining Death**. President's Commission for the Study of Ethical Problems in Medicine and Biomedical and Behavior Research, U.S. Government Printing Office, 1981.

• **Deciding to Forgo Life Sustaining Treatment**. President's Commission for the Study of Ethical Problems in Medicine and Biomedical and Behavior Research, U.S. Government Printing Office, 1983.

• James Rachels, **The End of Life**. Oxford University Press, 1986.

• Paul Ramsey, **Ethics at the Edges of Life**. Yale University Press, 1980.

• Tom Regan, **Matters of Life and Death: New Introductory Essays in Moral Philosophy**, 2nd ed. Random House, 1986.

• David H. Smith and Robert M. Veatch, eds., **Guidelines on the Termination of Life-Sustaining Treatment and the Care of the Dying**. Indiana University Press, 1987.

• **The Physician and the Hopelessly Ill Patient: Legal, Medical and Ethical Guidelines**. Society for the Right to Die, 1985.

• Robert M. Veatch, **Death, Dying, and the Biological Revolution: Our Last Quest for Responsibility**. Yale University Press, 1989.

• Robert F. Weir, ed., **Ethical Issues in Death and Dying**, 2nd ed. Columbia University Press, 1986.

Perinatal/Neonatal Issues

• Helga Kuhse and Peter Singer, **Should the Baby Live?** Oxford University Press, 1985.

• Jeff Lying, **Playing God in the Nursery**. W.W. Norton, 1985.

• Thomas H. Murray and Arthur L. Caplan, **Which Babies Shall Live? Humanistic Dimensions of the Care of Imperiled Newborns**. Humana Press, 1985.

• Earl E. Shelp, **Born to Die? Deciding the Fate of Critically Ill Newborns**. Oxford University Press, 1984.

• Robert F. Weir, **Selective Non-Treatment of Handicapped Newborns**. Oxford University Press, 1984.

Allocation of Healthcare Services

- Robert H. Blank, **Life, Death and Public Policy**. Northern Illinois University Press, 1988.
- Daniel Callahan, **Setting Limits: Medical Goals in an Aging Society**. Simon and Schuster, 1987.
- Larry R. Churchill, **Rationing Health Care in America**. University of Notre Dame Press, 1987.
- Norman Daniels, **Am I My Parents' Keeper? An Essay on Justice Between the Young and the Old**. Oxford University Press, 1988.
- Norman Daniels, **Just Health Care**. Cambridge University Press, 1985.
- Karen Lebacqz, **Six Theories of Justice**. Augsburg Publishing House, 1986.
- Alasdair MacIntyre, **Whose Justice? Which Rationality?** University of Notre Dame Press, 1988.
- **Securing Access to Health Care**. President's Commission for the Study of Ethical Problems in Medicine and Biomedical and Behavior Research, U.S. Government Printing Office, 1983.
- Charles B. Rosenberg, **Care of Strangers: The Rise of America's Hospital System**. Basic Books, 1987.
- Earl E. Shelp, **Justice and Health Care**. D. Reidel, 1981.
- Robert M. Veatch, **The Foundations of Justice: Why the Retarded and the Rest of Us Have Claims to Equality**. Oxford University Press, 1986.
- Gerald Winslow, **Triage and Justice**. University of California Press, 1989.

Morality, Theology and Medical Ethics

- Stanley Hauerwas, **Suffering Presence: Theological Reflections on Medicine, The Mentally Retarded, and the Church**. University of Notre Dame Press, 1986.
- Stephen E. Lammers and Allen Verhey, eds., **On Moral Medicine**. William B. Eerdmans Publishing Co., 1987.
- Martin E. Marty and Kenneth L. Vaux, eds., **Health/Medicine and the Faith Traditions**. The Park Ridge Center, 1989.
- Ronald L. Numbers and Darrel W. Amundsen, **Caring and Curing**. Macmillan Publishing Company, 1986.
- Earl E. Shelp, ed., **Theology and Bioethics: Exploring the Foundations and Frontiers**. Kluwer Academic Press, 1985.

Developmental and Gender Differences in Ethical Thinking

- Ronald Duska and Mariellen Whelan, **Moral Development, A Guide to Piaget and Kohlberg.** Paulist Press, 1975.
- Carol Gilligan, **In a Different Voice.** Harvard University Press, 1986.
- William G. Perry, Jr., **Forms of Intellectual and Ethical Development in the College Years.** Holt, Rinehart and Winston, Inc., 1968.